SAS ACTIVE LIBRARY

EMERGENCY
MEDIC

Barry Davies BEM

 HarperCollins*Publishers*

HarperCollins Publishers
Westerhill Rd, Bishopbriggs Glasgow G64 2QT

www.**fire**and**water**.co.uk

First published 2001

Reprint 10 9 8 7 6 5 4 3 2 1 0

© Barry Davies 2001

ISBN 0 00 710230 5

Picture credits: all images © HarperCollins, except for pp.23, 25, 26, 27, 29, 35, 37, 51, 54, 60, 61, 75, 77, 91, 93 (bottom), 94, 96 (bottom), 97 (top), 98, 99, 101, 199, 200, 201 © PS5 Ltd; pp. 56, 64, 84, 86, 87, 114, 122, 129, 131, 132, 144, 147, 149, 153, 154, 156, 161, 172, 192, 206, 207, 214, 215, 218, 219, 220 (top), 221 © Barry Davies ; pp.127, 151, 164, 168, 203, 212 © PhotoDisc; pp.168, 176, 177, 178, 179, 180, 196 © The Printer's Devil; pp. 167, © Edwin Moore; pp. 128, 148, 159, 230 © BCB Intrnational; p. 202 © Corbis; pp. 173, 189, 190 © Corel; p. 16 © Imperial War Museum.

Printed in Hong Kong by Midas

Contents

Burns

Diseases

Food & Water Contamination Diseases

Environmental Medical Problems

Dangerous Wildlife

Evacuation & Rescue

Travel Preparation & Planning

Medical Packs

Notes

Casualty Control

This Casualty Control chart maps out the essential actions or treatment required when you are faced with a medical emergency. It is intended to minimise the time between finding a casualty (or casualties) and deciding what steps you need to take to preserve life.

Work through each of the Actions until the casualty or casualties are in a stable condition. Cross references refer to the appropriates sections of the book which expand upon the recommended action in detail.

Action

➤ Check for your own and the casualty's safety

➤ Approach the casualty with care

➤ Evaluate the situation (see p.19)

Backup

➤ Communicate your problems to an appropriate agency as soon as is practical

➤ Designate any available help at the scene

Casualties

➤ For **INDIVIDUAL CASUALTIES** go to **ACTION 1** (see p.7)

➤ For **MULTIPLE CASUALTIES** first go to **ACTION 8** (see p.10)

➤ For **ENVIRONMENTAL CASUALTIES** (e.g. those affected by extremes of heat or cold) go to **ACTION 9** (see p.10)

➤ For **EVACUATION** go to **ACTION 10** (see p.11)

ACTION 1 ASSESS

Check if the casualty is

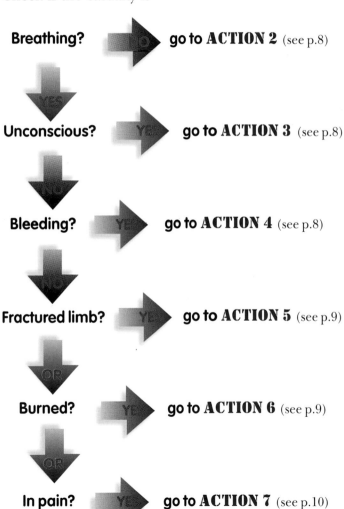

Breathing? NO **go to ACTION 2** (see p.8)

Unconscious? YES **go to ACTION 3** (see p.8)

Bleeding? YES **go to ACTION 4** (see p.8)

Fractured limb? YES **go to ACTION 5** (see p.9)

Burned? YES **go to ACTION 6** (see p.9)

In pain? YES **go to ACTION 7** (see p.10)

ACTION 2 ABC REGIME

➤ Perform the ABC regime immediately (see p.22)

➤ Ensure no pulse is evident before starting CPR

➤ Check for recovery signs (see p.29)

Continuing difficulty in breathing?

➤ Check for deeper airway obstruction

➤ Sucking wound to chest (see p.77)

➤ Crushed chest or broken ribs (see p.95)

➤ Consider cricothyroidotomy as a last resort (see p.39)

ACTION 3 RECOVERY

➤ If casualty is breathing but unconcious, place them in the recovery position (see p.30)

➤ Keep warm

➤ Continue ACTION 4 through to ACTION 10

ACTION 4 BLEEDING

➤ Use direct pressure (see p.59)

➤ Do not remove foreign objects - pad before dressing

➤ Use dressing to cover the wound

➤ Use second dressing if necessary

➤ Secure dressing

➤ Elevate limb   (contd)

If bleeding continues

➤ Apply indirect pressure (see p.61)

➤ Apply tourniquet if all else fails (see p.63) - consider **ACTION 10**

➤ Prevent shock (see p.68)

ACTION 5 FRACTURES

➤ Check for obvious signs: pain, deformity, and swelling

➤ Has the fracture caused a wound? - go to **ACTION 4**

➤ Splint the limb (see p.91)

➤ Is there pain? - go to **ACTION 7**

➤ Consider **ACTION 10**

➤ Prevent shock (see p.68)

ACTION 6 BURNS

➤ Use cold water to elevate burn damage

➤ Lightly cover burnt area with dressing

➤ Do not burst burn blisters

➤ Is there pain - go to **ACTION 7**

➤ Is the burnt area larger than two hand palms - consider **ACTION 10**

➤ Prevent shock (see p.68)

ACTION 7 PAIN RELIEF

➤ Use aspirin for less painful injuries

➤ Reassure the casualty

➤ Give restricted pain-killing drugs only under the direction of a qualified medical practitioner

ACTION 8 MULTIPLES

Assess all casualties before commencing any treatment for:

➤ Breathing

➤ Circulation

➤ Bleeding

➤ Body mass loss

➤ Consciousness

Prioritise urgency of treatment

➤ Begin individual treatment - go to ACTION 1

ACTION 9 CLIMATE

If the casualty been exposed to

Cold conditions:

➤ Check for other injuries - ACTION 1

➤ Place in sleeping bag

➤ Provide shelter

➤ Use body heat of second person

➤ Warm drinks if conscious

Hot conditions:

➤ Check for other injuries - **ACTION 1**

➤ Place in shade

➤ Remove heavy clothing

➤ Place cold/wet compress to the neck

➤ Replace fluids

Wet conditions:

➤ Check for other injuries -**ACTION 1**

➤ Shelter from wind

➤ Replace wet clothing with dry

➤ Place in sleeping bag

➤ Give warm drinks if conscious

ACTION 10 EVACUATE

Evacuate as a priority if the casualty is affected by any of the following:

➤ Breathing difficulties

➤ Heart attack

➤ Sever bleeding (external or suspected internal)

➤ The casualty remains unresponsive

➤ A tourniquet has been used

➤ Major limb fractures or spinal damage

➤ A known disease

WARNING

In all medical emergencies, the first priority is to make every effort to secure professional medical assistance. The procedures described in this book are designed to deal with medical emergencies when such professional help is unavailable or is delayed and the risk of death or long-term disablement to a casualty is immediate. Additionally, certain treatments should only be carried out when the casualty's life is undeniably threatened, and there is absolutely no chance of getting professional help. In all cases, calmness, common sense and general consensus, including that of the casualty when conscious, must prevail.

This book is not intended to be a comprehensive first aid manual but rather a guide to essential life-saving procedures and techniques for outdoor situations when no other medical help is readily available. All local laws, regulations and protocols should be taken into consideration by every helper *before* commencing upon emergency care.

The publishers cannot accept any responsibility for any prosecutions or proceedings brought or instituted against any person or body as a result of the use or misuse of any techniques described in this book, or any loss, injury or damage caused thereby.

Introduction

In general, there are five main threats to life:

➤ the inability to breathe
➤ severe blood loss
➤ heart malfunction
➤ shock
➤ disease

The first four can bring death within minutes but the latter can take from days to several weeks to develop. In many cases a death will be due to a combination of some of these threats.

However, the human body is extremely resilient, and is capable of surviving what may seem extensive and irreparable damage. Provided the heart is beating, and the lungs are functioning, there is always a chance of sustaining life. Blood loss can be stemmed and replaced, wounds can be closed, and infection or disease can be treated.

A medical emergency can happen at any time and if you are in an isolated or hostile area and without the means of immediate rescue, then your only resources are experience and a good medical pack. This pocket book is designed for just such an emergency. It is based broadly on the principles employed by SAS medics to preserve life in whatever dangerous or extreme environment they are in until the casualty can be extracted and hospitalised. Inevitably, *Emergency Medic* has its limitations, in terms of both content and subject depth but I hope it will provide you with the key skills to enable you to handle whatever emergency confronts you with confidence. Techniques for the expedient evacuation of a casualty are often missing from field medical books; however, rapid transportation to a safe medical facility truly does save lives. This theory has underpinned many a military campaign: soldiers know that there is a good chance of being wounded in battle but they also know that the military medical system has a good chance of keeping them alive providing they can reach a proper medical facility swiftly. This holds true for any medical emergency and for this reason, I place great emphasis on rescue and evacuation techniques.

THE THREAT TO LIFE

It is often said that we can live without food for four weeks, water for four days and air for four minutes. I am not so sure about the duration for food and water, but the air estimation is certainly correct. The brain needs oxygen and when confronted with a casualty the first thing to look for are signs of life – that the casualty is breathing and that a pulse is detectable. The first tells us the airway is clear and the second that blood is circulating around the body – together they tell us there is hope.

The next problem, both for the medic and the casualty, is fear. Fear is an instinctive reaction for anyone faced with the uncertain, especially where there is an immediate threat to life. Behaviour and reaction are always influenced by fear, as are the prospects for obtaining help. Fear can make people react irrationally, which can be dangerous when handling casualties.

It is always best to explain the situation in a calm, optimistic and confident manner. If you are part of a group, keep everyone involved and busy at all levels, from planning a rescue to helping with the casualty – idleness will only give time to reflect on any fears or discomfort. Acceptance of fear as a natural reaction to any threatening situation will produce two immediate and positive benefits:

➤ You will be able to dismiss the fear of being afraid, which is often a burden in itself. True courage may be found in people who freely admit to fear, but still go on to do their best in the circumstances they face.

➤ You will find yourself more likely to be able to carry out considered rather than uncoordinated actions. You will recognise that there is always something that can be done to improve the situation.

SAS MEDICS

SAS medics are highly trained personnel who under-go a medical course at the SAS base at Hereford prior to attending one of several hospitals where they help to treat actual patients. SAS medics are trained to deal with everything from childbirth to massive gunshot injuries and to work in the crudest of conditions. They are equipped with a pack that supports this training and which allows them to prescribe a range of medications and drugs plus carry out minor surgery. This ability to carry out life-saving first aid and deal with most medical situations is of enormous value to a four-man patrol operating behind the enemy lines. In many such cases, an injured soldier

An SAS medic at work

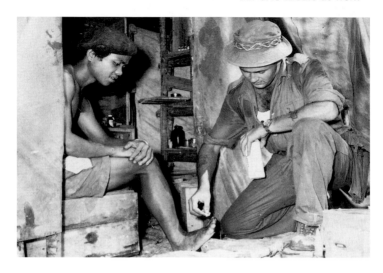

would have no prospect of receiving friendly assistance and the patrol medic will be totally responsible for his well-being. However, SAS medics are not doctors; they are simply soldiers who have received limited, although highly advanced, training in life-saving techniques.

The Excursion Medic

Any excursion into the wilderness or uninhabited areas of the world requires that a basic medical pack should be carried and that someone in the party should possess the knowledge to use its contents effectively. When such a touring party comprises four or more people, then at least one of these should be medically qualified. In the event of a medical emergency, that person will be deemed responsible for the

SAS ACTION

➤ During my 18 years service with the SAS, I witnessed our patrol medics saving the lives of several of their comrades. In two such cases the injuries looked horrendous yet the patients made a quick and full recovery. In the first instance two unqualified signallers were double feeding a mortar during a fire-fight, which resulted in the premature explosion of a mortar bomb. One man lost his eye and right hand up to the mid-wrist section. In another similar incident, the backblast of a rocket launcher totally removed the right arm of a soldier from the shoulder down. In both cases, SAS medics stemmed the bleeding, prevented shock and kept the casualties alive until they could be airlifted to hospital. In spite of their horrific injuries, both men made a full recovery, thanks to the prompt and confident actions of the medics.

medical well-being of the party; throughout this book, this 'medically responsible person' is referred to as the medic. In larger groups where several medically trained people may be available, the primary responsibility will rest with the most highly qualifed individual which, in descending order, would normally be

➤ doctor

➤ paramedic

➤ nurse

➤ trained first aid personnel

➤ team leader (no experience)

Knowledge of first aid skills, however basic, is valuable even in everyday life, but when you are confronted with a serious casualty in the wilderness, such knowledge becomes immeasurably important. Even when medical training and equipment is limited, or totally non-existent, it is still possible to save life if you know the basic principles of first aid.

Emergency Action

EVALUATION: GENERAL RULES

Always make a quick appraisal of what has happened. Do not approach an injured person unless you are absolutely sure there is no danger to yourself or others. For example, if a rockslide has occurred partially covering the casualty, more rocks may fall. If the casualty is clear of risk, approach and render assistance. If the prevailing situation continues to present further dangers to life, you should carefully remove the casualty to safe ground before checking for injury.

Casualties in danger

Much is made of spinal injuries (see Back Injury, p. 100) and that a casualty who has fallen must not be moved. Unless you have physical evidence of a spinal injury, e.g. the casualty has fallen from a height or received a head injury, and there is a prevailing risk, then the casualty should be moved to safety without undue delay. Remember to lift with great care, keeping the head in natural line with the body (see p. 100).

PRIORITISING CASUALTIES

In most cases medical emergencies will be hopefully limited to individuals. However, there is always the possibility that several people have been injured at the same time. The first task in any medical emergency is to establish a process of prioritisation of the wounded. Casualties are generally sorted into categories.

Those who require urgent assistance to prevent immediate death, e.g. those suffering from respiratory and circulatory disorders must be given priority, and those who have suffered major body-mass loss which results in severe haemorrhaging will also require immediate attention. A major disaster may well cause some casualties to be hopelessly wounded, putting them beyond recovery from any immediate assistance. In such a case the medic must identify such injuries and assess how long the casualty will live without assistance, and if assistance is given, will it prove beneficial. While formulating your priorities, keep the following rules in mind.

EMERGENCY PRIORITIES

➤ Exclude taking any action that will put you in danger. If you become injured then you will be in no position to help anyone else.

➤ Do not panic, no matter how serious the situation may look. Take several deep breaths to calm yourself, act professionally, offer hope and encouragement.

(Cont'd)

➤ Individual casualties will need to be assessed as to their injuries. For this you will need to use all your senses – ask (if the casualty is conscious), look (and if possible feel over the body for broken bones, blood etc), listen, smell – think and act.

➤ If the casualty is conscious, they will be an important source of information. Ask them what happened and to describe their symptoms.

➤ Think about your actions first then act quickly and carefully. Boost the morale of your casualty. Offer comfort and reassurance thus building the casualty's mental strength to live.

➤ If there are any other uninjured survivors, get them to help you in any way they can. Always ask (out of earshot of any injured person) if anyone has any medical experience.

➤ Separate as soon as possible those who are saveable

MEDICAL EMERGENCIES: PRIORITY ACTIONS

To repeat the point stated above, in any emergency situation, your first and most immediate concerns should be the casualty's ability to breath and whether their heart is beating. In dealing with these points under pressure, it is useful to memorise and rehearse the steps of the ABC regime:

Airway, Breathing, Circulation.

Airway: Check for Breathing

If the casualty is talking, then their airway is open and breathing will not be impaired. To determine if an unconscious casualty is breathing, listen with your ear close to the casualty's nose and mouth. You should be able to hear and feel any breath. Watch out for chest and abdominal movement at the same time. If there is no sign of breathing, you must take immediate action to ensure that the casualty's air passage is clear.

If the injured person is unconscious, it may be that their airway is blocked by the position of their head, which causes the tongue to fall back in the mouth and seal the airway (right).

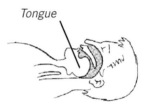

Tongue

To remedy this, use either a chin lift or a jaw thrust:

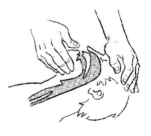

➤ **Chin lift:** place the fingers of one hand under the jaw and gently lift it upwards to bring the chin forward. To open the mouth, use the thumb of the same hand to depress the lower lip lightly. The thumb may also be placed behind the lower teeth and, simultaneously, the chin gently lifted.

➤ **Jaw thrust:** grasp the angles of the jaw bone, one hand on each side, and move the jaw forward.

Care must be taken at all times not to move the neck.

If there is still no breathing, there may be an obstruction in the airway.

To clear an airway obstruction:

➤ Use a suction device to remove vomit or secretions. However, if no such device is available, the airway takes priority over everything. Turn the casualty onto his side, trying as far as possible to keep the head in line with the rest of the body.

➤ Check quickly inside the mouth to find any other cause of blockage; remove any blockage, taking care not to push any object further into the mouth. If dentures are intact and not causing a blockage, keep them in place.

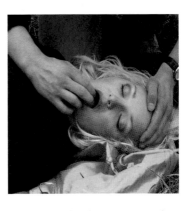

For dealing with more complicated blockages, see also the section on choking, p.34.

Once the air passage is open and clear, the casualty may begin breathing again. If this happens, and his heart is beating, put him into the recovery position (see p.30). Be alert to a visible injury to the front or back of the head which might indicate damage to the neck or spine. Improvise some form of head support to keep the head correctly positioned.

Breathing: Artificial Ventilation

Having checked the airway is clear, if breathing does not recommence, the casualty must be given help immediately. You must 'breathe' for them and this can best be done on a mouth-to-mouth basis (as described in the section on CPR below, see p.25). If the heart is beating and a pulse can be felt (see below), continue giving assisted breaths at a rate of between sixteen and eighteen a minute. When the casualty begins breathing for himself, continue giving assistance at his natural rate until breathing is normal and then place him in the recovery position (see p. 30).

If you are certain is no heartbeat, chest compression must be carried out as described below.

Circulation: Check for Heartbeat

Before starting any resuscitation it is important to check whether or not the casualty's heart is beating. Checking the casualty's pulse will determine whether the heart is still beating. This can be done in either of the following ways:

➤ Using the tips of two fingers, gently slide them down the side of the casualty's Adam's apple towards the back of the neck until you feel a soft groove. Press gently on this spot (pic. 1).

➤ Rest your fingers lightly on the front of the wrist, about 1 cm (0.5 inch) back from the wrist joint on the thumb side (close to where a watchstrap would normally fasten) (pic. 2).

➤ Check for 10 seconds (and up to a minute for severe hypothermia cases).

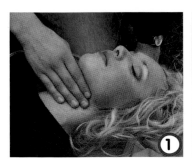
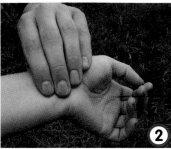

If there is no heartbeat, chest compression must be carried out as described below. This is often done in conjunction with artificial ventilation and, together, these processes are known as CPR (cardiopulmonary resuscitation).

WARNING

➤ BE SURE that there is **NO** heartbeat before beginning chest compression. Far more harm than good will be done if attempted chest compression interferes with an existing heartbeat, however weak.

CPR (CARDIOPULMONARY RESUSCITATION)

Artificial Ventilation

➤ Check breathing (look, listen, feel) and circulation response and ascertain required CPR action.

➤ Supporting the neck with one hand, ease the

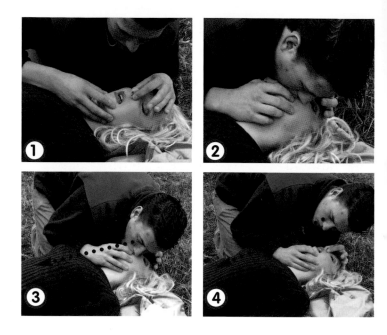

head backwards with the other. Keeping the head back, lift the chin upwards.

➤ Taking a deep breath, pinch the casualty's nose to prevent air loss (pic. 1), open your mouth wide and seal your lips around his open mouth (pic. 2).

➤ Blow into his lungs, watching for expansion of the chest (pic. 3). When the maximum expansion is reached, raise your head well clear and breathe out and in. Look now for the chest contraction (pic. 4).

➤ When this has happened, repeat the procedure once more. It may be more convenient to use mouth-to-nose contact. In this case, the casualty's mouth must be kept shut to prevent the loss of air.

➤ Following the two long assisted breaths check the carotid pulse in the neck. If breathing is absent but pulse is present, assist with rescue breathing (one breath every 5 seconds, about 12 breaths per minute). If there is no pulse, give cycles of 15 chest compressions (at a rate of around 80 to 100 compressions per minute) followed by two slow breaths.

Chest Compression

➤ Check that the casualty is lying on a firm surface.

➤ Kneeling alongside, locate the bottom of the breastbone. Measure the width of two fingers up and place the heel of one hand on the bone. Lay the other hand over the first (pic. 1).

➤ Keeping the elbows rigid, lean forward so that your arms are vertical and your weight bearing down on the casualty's chest (pic. 2).

➤ Depress the breastbone by between 4 and 5 cm (2–2¹/₂ inches). Lean back to release the

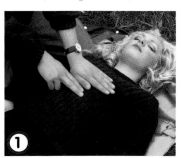
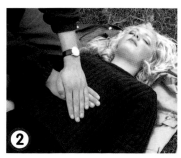

pressure, so allowing the breastbone to return to its original position.

➤ Perform 15 compressions at the rate of about 80 per minute. (Count, one back, two back, three back, and so on, leaning forward on each number.)

CPR By One Person

In normal conditions, breathing and circulation take place at the same time. The casualty needs both, so assisted breathing and chest compression must be carried out together. If you are alone, the procedures have to be alternated.

➤ As soon as the first 15 compressions have been given, restore the open air-passage position of the head and provide two more assisted breaths.

➤ When this has been done, continue this cycle: 15 compressions and two assisted breaths for a full minute.

➤ Continue the treatment, checking for heartbeat only if there are signs of improvement (e.g. the casualty breathes, moves or makes a noise).

CPR By Two People

If two people are available to help, one should first seek help if possible before assisting with CPR. However, with two people available, they should each provide part of the treatment, with one person assisting breathing and the other providing the compressions.

➤ At the start, give two assisted breaths (pic. 1)

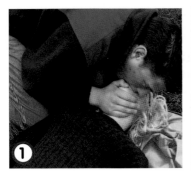
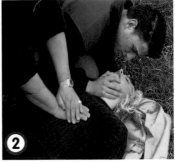

and follow these with five compressions (pic. 2). Then establish a pattern of two assisted breaths followed by fifteen compressions. Aim at a rate of one compression per second.

➤ Discontinue compression when the casualty recovers.

➤ Continue with assisted breathing until the casualty breathes for himself.

When breathing and heartbeat are both established, place him in the recovery position (see p.30) after checking for other injuries.

RECOVERY SIGNS

It is important to look for and recognise the recovery signs in casualties who are receiving CPR. The blueish colouring of the lips should slowly return to normal as will the facial skin tone. The pulse will return and the casualty may groan or start to move.

As the casualty recovers you will find resistance to your CPR efforts, indicating that spontaneous breathing has returned.

ABC PRIORITY CHECKLIST

➤ Breathing and conscious – check for injuries.

➤ Breathing and unconscious – place in recovery position if injuries allow.

➤ Not breathing but with chest and abdomen movement – check for airway blockage.

➤ Not breathing and with no sign of chest movement – start immediate resuscitation.

THE RECOVERY POSITION

Generally, an unconscious person who is breathing and who has a reasonable heartbeat, and is without other injuries demanding immediate attention should be put into the recovery (or coma) position.

This position, illustrated in the six pictures opposite, is the safest because it minimises the risk of impeded breathing. The tilted-back head ensures open air passages. The face-down attitude allows any vomit or other liquid obstruction to drain from the mouth. The spread of the limbs will maintain the body in its position. If fractures or other injuries prevent suitable placing of the limbs, use rolled clothing or other padded objects to prop the injured person in this position.

Where the casualty has a suspected spine injury, a special spinal recovery position should be used if there are sufficient helpers available (see p. 100).

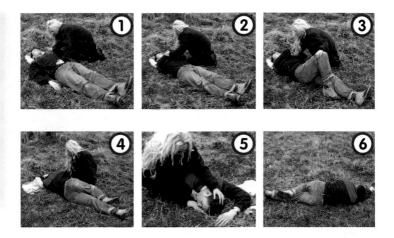

EMERGENCY CONDITIONS

Cardiac Arrest

A heart attack can occur at any time, anywhere and without warning and in many cases, it can be fatal. When the blood vessels that supply the heart (coronary arteries) become blocked it produces a heart attack.

The main symptoms of a heart attack are:

➤ a dull or heavy pain in the centre of the chest (primary)

➤ sweating, nausea or vomiting and breathlessness (secondary)

The pain is called angina which results when the heart muscle is starved of oxygen. It only takes 15–30 seconds to lose consciousness after the heart stops due to lack of oxygen to the brain after the blood pressure drops to zero. You may also encounter muscular spasms, like those of a fit and vomiting. The part of the heart which is deprived of blood dies rapidly, the effect of which is to produce a crushing pain in the centre of the chest. The damaged heart results in a weak rapid and irregular pulse and the casualty normally collapses.

Vagal inhibition and ventricular fibrillation

These conditions are possible reasons why a heart will stop beating. One of the functions of the vagus nerve is to control the heart rate. It controls the beating of the heart by keeping it at a steady pace. The heart would beat at approximately 100 beats per minute without it, but the vagus keeps the rate to approximately 60 beats per minute, when at rest, but adjusts effects by either slowing the heart considerably or stopping it altogether. The most likely reasons for this to happen are poor health, shock, either a physical pain or a nasty fright, pressure on a certain part of the neck, or by a direct blow to the front, lower chest.

Ventricular fibrillation is when the ventricles start beating at over 300 beats per minute due to an irritable piece of heart muscle. At this speed they cannot fill with blood and so the blood stops circulating. After three to four minutes, death will occur because the brain stops functioning. An irritable heart muscle is usually the result of a previous heart attack or if the person suffers from angina. An angina attack can sometimes act as a warning sign.

TREATMENT

Heart attacks must be treated without delay. Think quickly, stay calm and start resuscitation immediately. Once the heart has stopped beating you have only minutes before irreversible brain damage occurs unless you can restore the circulation to the brain. Resuscitation and cardiac massage should be started immediately. If after four minutes there is no response to CPR (p. 25) there is little chance that the heart will ever start again.

A casualty who remains breathing or responds to resuscitation should be placed in a prone position in order to lower the oxygen demand on the body. Search the person's pockets for any prescriptive heart medications. Give sublingual nitro-glycerine if available – three tablets, one each at five minute intervals – or asprin. Treat for pain and nausea as appropriate. Administer oxygen if available and arrange an immediate evacuation to a good medical facility as a priority. Continue to monitor respiration and pulse until evacuation can be arranged.

Unconsciousness

When a casualty is completely unaware of what is going on around them or is unable to make purposeful movements, they are deemed to be unconscious. People who faint are briefly unconscious while those in a coma are in continuing unconsciousness. If someone collapses or you find an unconscious person, try to establish the cause. Check the immediate area to ascertain it is safe before approaching the body. If someone has collapsed within a group, ask if someone noticed any prior indication of stress, such as feeling faint, chest pains. Has the casualty been drinking heavily or are they on medication? Is the casualty a known drug user? The most common causes of unconsciousness are stroke, head injury, drunkenness, poisoning and epilepsy.

TREATMENT

Using the ABC regime (see p.22), check breathing and circulation and carry out CPR as necessary. Try talking to the casualty: if there is no response, shake them a little, but do not move them needlessly. Next assess their reaction to pain by pinching the flesh sharply. After checking for injuries, place in the recovery position (p. 30) until they regain consciousness or evacuation can be arranged.

Choking

Choking is a serious condition requiring immediate assistance as the airway is blocked and therefore no air is getting through to the lungs.

CHOKING SYMPTOMS

➤ being suddenly unable to breathe or speak

➤ grabbing at the throat

➤ the skin turning pale blue

➤ In an unconscious person, listen for wheezing sounds, and check to see if the chest is rising.

TREATMENT

The first priority is to try and remove whatever is causing the blockage in the windpipe. If the casualty is conscious, try to get them to cough it up. If this does not work, make a visual check of the mouth to see if the object can be cleared with a finger. If not,

➤ Bend the casualty as far forward as possible, preferably so that the head is below the level of the lungs.

➤ Give five sharp slaps between the shoulder blades with the heel of the hand and check to see if the obstruction has been dislodged.

This usually is enough to remove the object, but if it does not work and choking persists, try to clear it by using abdominal thrusts:

➤ Stand behind the casualty and put your arms around them.

➤ Ball one fist and lock it in place with the palm of your other hand (pic 1), make sure that one thumb is pressing into the abdomen.

➤ Sharply pull the hands inwards under the ribs (pic 2).

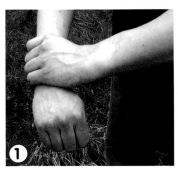
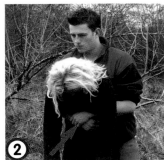

➤ Repeat up to four more times before checking whether the object has been expelled.

If this does not succeed at first, give five more back slaps and then five more abdominal thrusts. Keep trying until the object becomes dislodged. It is very unusual for this procedure not to work.

Choking and Unconscious

If the choking casualty becomes unconscious, first lie them on their side with their abdomen supported against your knee and give four to five back slaps. If this does not dislodge the object, turn them onto their back, kneel astride them and perform the abdominal thrusts (see below):

➤ Locate the heel of one hand just below the ribcage and cover it with the other hand.

➤ Press sharply inwards and upwards with the heel of the hand up to five times.

➤ Check in the mouth to see if the object has been expelled.

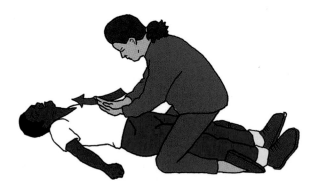

➤ Continue alternating back slaps with abdominal thrusts until the obstruction is removed.

If the casualty begins to breathe normally, place them in the recovery position (p. 30) and check breathing and pulse rates every three minutes. If breathing does not recommence and/or there is no pulse, start immediately on the ABC regime with assisted breathing and, if necessary, chest compressions.

Self-Help on Choking

If you find that you are alone and choking, find something like a post or a tree trunk and push it inwards and upwards into your abdomen to expel the air, and hopefully, the object. You could also attempt to use your own hands made into a fist to achieve the same effect.

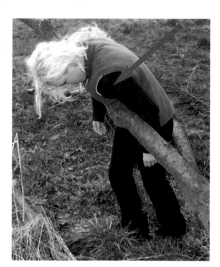

Cricothyroidotomy

The above procedures should, in most circumstances, remove any blockage from a person's throat. However, there may be occasions where they are unsuccessful and more radical treatment is required: cutting into the choking person's throat below the blockage, using a technique known as cricothyroidotomy. (This can also be used where a substantial injury to the jaw area prevents the patient from breathing.)

You will require the following:

➤ A sharp, narrow blade (e.g. a scalpel or a penknife)

➤ A short hollow tube (a ballpoint pencase, tubing from a backpack and small syringes have all been used

➤ Some means of sterilising the above (boiling water or a flame); however, do not waste time on this if it is likely to cause a delay

The casualty, if conscious, will be very active and difficult to restrain. It is vital that you focus his attention on what must be done in order to facilitate air into the lungs in a calm but assertive manner. Carry out the following procedure with swiftness and confidence.

➤ Place the casualty on the ground with their shoulders slightly raised by a folded towel or something similar, allowing the head to fall back slightly and extending the throat. If available, get others to hold the head and shoulders still and continue to reassure the casualty.

➤ Run a finger down the Adam's apple on the front of the neck and find another small projection just below it. Between these two points on the throat, a central valley can be felt just beneath the skin (pics 1, 2).

➤ Use your thumb and forefinger to stretch and im-mobilise the skin around this area with one hand.

➤ Make a horizontal incision over midpoint of the central valley (pic. 3). The incision should be small and pushed straight down for about 1–2 cm ($^1/_2$ –$^3/_4$ in). The blade should move easily as it cuts through the windpipe.

➤ Turn the scalple upside down and twist the handle sideways to widen the cut until a finger-sized hole is obtained.

➤ The moment the airway is open you should hear the casualty gasping as the air is sucked in. Use your fingers to enlarge the opening and allow the casualty to fill their lungs. Continue to reassure the casualty.

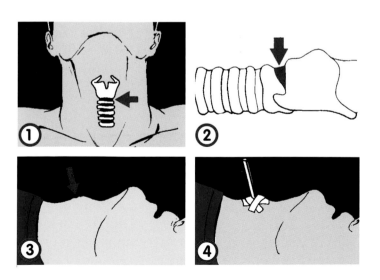

➤ Once the casualty starts to relax, insert the tube into the opening and secure it with adhesive tape, plasters or bandages to prevent it from being sucked in or dislodged from the opening (pic. 4). If the tube is narrow, you may have to assist the casualty's breathing by blowing air into the lungs via the tube and sucking out CO_2.

➤ If after completing a successful cricothyroid-otomy the casualty is still not breathing, then apply artificial ventilation (see p.25) to the airway. Once breathing normally, place the casualty in a comfortable position.

➤ Continue to check breathing and pulse while waiting for evacuation.

Drowning

Drowning is defined as death resulting from suffoca-tion caused by total (mouth and nose) submersion in water for a duration long enough to stop the heart. In the wilderness, drowning normally results because of several factors: diving in shallow water, the inability to swim properly, and being swept away by strong and dangerous currents. Many drowning accidents can be avoided if caution is exercised and proper procedures are strictly adhered to while near to or crossing water. If someone is in difficulty in water, swim or wade out to them as quickly as possible. While supporting the floating body, remove any obstructions from the air-way and begin mouth-to-mouth resuscitation (see p.25); this should start while still in the water and continue as you move towards dry land. When ashore, place the casualty on a firm surface and check breath-ing and heartbeat – continue with CPR (see p.25) for as long as required. Do not worry about getting the casualty to heave up any swallowed water. Once spontaneous breathing has returned, place the casualty in the recovery position (p.30) and cover with a blanket. If the water is very cold, check for hypothermia (see p.156). Continue to monitor the casualty every 10 minutes until they are evacuated.

Carbon Monoxide (CO) Poisoning

Carbon monoxide gas is produced by the incomplete combustion of fuel and outdoors, is most often associated with cooking stoves. In an unventilated area, such as the interior of a tent, it can quickly become lethal, causing death by asphyxia within 15 to 20 minutes. A major problem is that the gas is odourless, colourless and tasteless, which makes it difficult to detect.

CO POISONING SYMPTOMS

➤ Headache

➤ Bounding pulse

➤ Dilated pupils

➤ The skin, especially the lips, may deepen in colour to cherry pink

➤ Confusion, and impaired breathing

➤ In the advanced stages, unconsciousness may occur. The same degree of poisoning may affect individuals sharing accommodation with differing degrees of the same symptoms. This variation in individuals is a classic sign of carbon monoxide poisoning.

TREATMENT

For those suspected of carbon monoxide poisoning the best treatment is to maximise oxygenation, that is, get them into the fresh air. If anyone is unconscious but breathing normally, place them in the recovery position (p.30). Where breathing has stopped, follow the ABC regime (see p.22) and start CPR if required. Give 100 per cent oxygen if available. Evacuate to a medical facility where high oxygen absorption can be provided more efficiently. Where evacuation is delayed, monitor the casualty's breathing, pulse and responsiveness at 10-minute intervals. Remove everyone from the area of contamination and extinguish the source of the carbon monoxide.

However, prevention is better than cure so the following guidelines should always be followed:

➤ Always ensure good ventilation if using an oil-burning stove.

➤ Check any manufactured stove, and maintain its clean running.

➤ Always turn off or extinguish any petrol or aviation-type stove before going to sleep.

Childbirth

Procedure

If not already resting, get the mother to a safe, quiet place. Place some support behind her back and shoulders so that she is as comfortable as possible. Respect the woman's choice of delivery position (this is not always on their back and can include kneeling or

AUTHOR'S NOTE

➤ It is unlikely that a heavily pregnant woman will go trekking off into the wilderness but you may well find yourself somewhere in the world having to assist a woman in labour. Childbirth is not a serious medical condition and in the vast majority of cases presents no problems. Where help is required, the medically responsible person should offer their services, but they should never intrude. Certain cultures are very wary of strangers viewing their womenfolk.

squatting). Remove any clothing that may impede the childbirth. Wash you hands for at least four minutes, cleaning your nails in the process. To further prevent infection, wear surgical gloves if available.

You should have a clean blanket or towel ready in order to wrap the baby after delivery. You will also need sterile ligatures and scissors with which to tie and cut the umbilical cord. If ligatures are not available, cut five pieces (25 cm/10 inches long) of string, cord or even laces and boil them for at least ten minutes.

A sudden rush of fluid indicates the amniotic sac around the baby in the womb has ruptured. When the baby's head appears at the vaginal opening support it with your cupped hand. The baby is under great pressure from the mother's contractions but do not allow him or her to 'shoot out' as this can cause the mother's peroneal area (immediately below the vagina) to tear. Likewise, do not pull or twist the baby's head as it emerges. The baby should slide out naturally without assistance. Once the head is clear, it will twist to one side facing the mother's thigh thus allowing the shoulders and arms to emerge easily.

If any of the amniotic sac is covering the baby's face then this should be torn as soon as possible to prevent asphyxia.

Support the baby as it emerges. Once the head is clear check to make sure that the umbilical cord has not become entangled around the baby's neck. If this is the case, carefully unwind it. (Never pull the cord during or after the delivery as it is still attached to the mother.) Once the baby has totally emerged, hold it face down and remove any fluid or membrane from around the nose and mouth.

Lift the baby clear, being very careful as newborn babies are very slippery, and pass the baby to the mother. Do not cut the umbilical cord at this stage. Wrap the baby in the clean sheet or towel, taking care to cover the head while leaving the face exposed. The baby may start to cry although many simply breathe in a normal restful manner. If normal breathing is not detected soon after it is born then flick the soles of the baby's feet with your finger. Alternatively, rub the baby's back to stimulate breathing. (Do not smack the baby.) If there is no response or the baby's face becomes blue, begin resuscitation immediately.

If evacuation to a medical facility has been organised then there is no need to cut the umbilical cord. The placenta (or afterbirth) usually emerges about 10–15 minutes after the baby is born. This can be placed in a plastic bag and sent to hospital with the mother and child for further examination.

In the event that no evacuation is immediately possible or given that the cord is very short, it may become necessary to cut the cord. This should not be done until the afterbirth has been delivered and the cord has stopped pulsating. If you are unsure wait at least 15 minutes.

Using the ligatures or sterilised string make two ties, one 15 cm (6 inches) from the baby's stomach and another at 20 cm (8 inches). Cut the cord with sterile scissors. Dress the end of the cord still attached to the baby. Check for bleeding; if none is detected then place a second ligature some 10cm from the baby's stomach. Lay the cord against the baby's bellybutton and cover with a sterile dressing.

Note: the ligatures must be tied very tight to prevent bleeding.

Breech Delivery

When the baby's position inside the womb is reversed, that is, it is resting head up, then a breech delivery will occur. This means the baby will emerge feet first. As with a normal birth, support the baby, but allow it to hang from the birth canal during delivery. Do not try to force the baby out. However, if after the shoulders have emerged the head is retained for more than three minutes you will be required to assist. Grasp the baby's feet and lift the body gently over the mother's abdomen. Lift, do not pull. This should free the mouth and nose and release the head. Continue the delivery as normal.

Ruptured Appendix (Peritonitis)

Appendicitis is the inflammation and possible infection of the appendix, a small finger-like extension of the colon. It is an illness than can occur at any time to even the healthiest of individuals. Although this is not immediately a life-threatening condition, in the

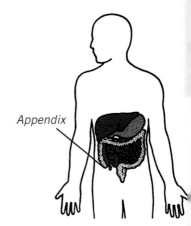

Appendix

APPENDICITIS SYMPTOMS

➤ Intermittent pain around the belly. Some hours later (6–24 hours) as the pain increases, it is confined to the right lower quarter of the abdomen. It is this shift in pain that usually indicates appendicitis.

(Cont'd)

➤ Casualty usually tries to lie still and avoid movement which accentuates the pain, with knees drawn up to the chest

➤ Tenderness to touch in the lower right quarter

➤ Intermittent vomiting

➤ Pain and tenderness felt throughout the entire abdominal area indicates that the appendix may have ruptured

➤ Check if there has been any history of diarrhoea, as this may indicate that the pain is not appendicitis; however, assess this as only part of the range of presenting symptoms

wilderness, it may take some time to organise proper treatment by which time, the appendix may have ruptured to spread infection throughout the whole abdominal cavity (peritonitis). Pain is accompanied by a high fever, normally in excess of 38°C (101°F).

TREATMENT

Providing the casualty can be evacuated quickly to a medical facility where surgery can be performed, there is little or no problem, however in the wilderness this is not always possible. Lay the casualty down in the most comfortable position for them and keep warm. Give no food although small amounts of water should be given from time to time to avoid dehydration. Treat for pain and nausea until an evacuation can be arranged.

Amputation

Accidental amputations of a digit or limb represents a serious problem because of severe blood loss and shock. Depending on the severity of the wound, the priority is to control the bleeding and remove the patient to a proper medical facility as soon as possible.

Where the limb, finger or toe has been severed and not crushed, there is always the possibility of re-attachment. Secure the severed part as cleanly as possible and dispatch it with the patient. Make a note of the time the amputation occurred.

TREATMENT

➤ Perform the ABC regime (p.22) as necessary. Breathing and pulse should be constantly monitored and the casualty resuscitated if necessary.

➤ Slow the bleeding by applying direct pressure (see p.59) to the main artery immediately above the stump or if this is not possible, pad the stump itself. The immediate padding should be sterile, but if the bleeding is severe then speed is more important and any clean cloth will suffice. Make sure the padding is tight.

➤ If the bleeding persists place a second and third dressing over the original.

➤ Once the bleeding is controlled, the casualty should be rested with the feet elevated in order to maintain an adequate blood supply to the head and body.

➤ Treat for shock.

SAVING THE LIMB

➤ Wrap the severed limb in a clean cover and place in a clean plastic bag or waterproof container.

➤ Keep in a cool place (e.g. in a second container sitting on ice or snow) but do not cover directly with ice or chilled water.

➤ Evacuate the limb with the patient and record the time of the accident.

POST EMERGENCY

Once the casualty has been stabilised, i.e. they are breathing on their own and their circulation has been restored, it is time to make a more detailed observation. Start making some notes and record the vital signs.

Checking Vital Signs

While the vital signs will not necessarily tell you what's wrong, they will let you know how the casualty is responding to any trauma. It is important to note and record any changes in the vital signs:

State of consciousness

Is the casualty alert and able to communicate normally? If there is no response to verbal stimulation, do they react to physical stimulation, such as pinching? Is the casualty totally unconscious?

Respiration

Is the breathing normal (12–18 breaths per minute)?
Is the breathing shallow or deep? Is there any noise
associated with their breathing?

Pulse

The pulse rate should be around 60–80 per minute.
While you are checking feel for the rhythm and quality. The beat should be even and strong. See p.24 on
how to check a pulse.

Skin

Always check skin colouring because changes are frequently caused by the amount of blood reaching the
skin surface. If more blood is allowed to the surface,
then the skin will redden or flush, which could be a
sign of fever. If less blood is allowed to the surface,
the skin will become white, indicating that there
could be internal bleeding, shock or hypothermia. A
blue tinge to the skin points towards lack of oxygen,
while a yellow skin points to liver failure or infection.

Your examination and recording of the vital signs,
together with what the casualty can tell you, will help
you establish the required priority of treatment. Some
symptoms will be more obvious and immediate (broken leg or heart attack) while others will not be so
apparent (internal bleeding or disease).

The Examination

The most logical way to start the examination of a
casualty is from the head down. If conscious, talk to
him or her as you carry out an examination; ask them

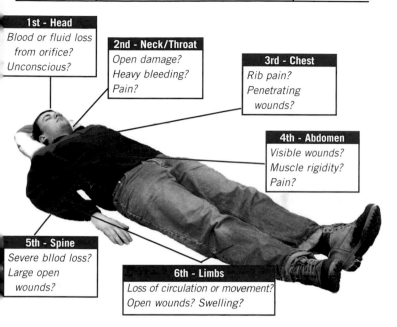

1st - Head
Blood or fluid loss
from orifice?
Unconscious?

2nd - Neck/Throat
Open damage?
Heavy bleeding?
Pain?

3rd - Chest
Rib pain?
Penetrating
wounds?

4th - Abdomen
Visible wounds?
Muscle rigidity?
Pain?

5th - Spine
Severe bllod loss?
Large open
wounds?

6th - Limbs
Loss of circulation or movement?
Open wounds? Swelling?

questions but make sure they are not leading. Rather than 'Were you unconscious for five minutes or less?' it would be be 'Could you estimate how long you were unconscious?' Make a mental note of the more serious injuries as you progress.

Head

Check the head for bleeding or fluid loss; is the blood from a cut or contusion or from an orifice such as the nose, ears, eyes or mouth? Has the casualty been unconscious, even for a few seconds? Do they feel any dizziness etc.?

Neck

Examine the neck for signs of physical damage. Use your fingers to gently feel the spine from the shoulders up to the base of the skull – record any pain. Check for any open damage to the sides of the neck and the throat – excessive bleeding from large cuts or deep penetrations.

Chest

Use your open palms to gently compress the ribs on both sides – check for pain. Look for any cuts or contusions, especially deep penetrating wounds.

Abdomen

Spread your palm and gently press down on the abdomen. Cup the hipbones with the palms of your hand and push down then pull back towards the body centreline. Check for visible wounds, contusions, muscle rigidity and pain.

Spine

Push your flat palm under the casualty and feel along the spine with your fingers. Check for any severe blood loss or large open wound.

Limbs

Individually check each arm and leg from top to bottom by gently sliding both hands down the surface. Check for open wounds, swelling, bleeding, lack of circulation or motion.

Upon completion of a full examination you must decide whether the casualty can be treated at the present location, and if there is there a medic available, do they have the required skill and equipment? If not, then the casualty will have to be moved and/or an evacuation arranged (see p.191).

AUTHOR'S NOTE

➤ It is always a good idea to carry some form of medical record with you. There are several ways of doing this such as a bracelet or medallion, but by far the best is a single sheet of paper with a brief medical history typed on it. This should be kept in a waterproof sleeve in your wallet or a secure pocket. It should contain vital details of your medical history, such as serious disease, operations, any drug sensitivity or allergy and blood group. This information can be of great value if you happen to become unconscious.

Checking a Pulse

A normal pulse rate is around 65–70 beats per minute. The resting pulse, taken when we first awaken, is normally a little lower. This resting pulse rate falls the fitter we become. In real terms this means the heart rate of an unfit person doing exercise will be around 120 beats per minute; with the same exercise in a fit person it will be greatly reduced to around 85–90 beats per minute. In the course of a minute's activity the hearts of both the fit and unfit person will pump the same volume of blood, the difference being that the fit person's heart will need less beats to do it.

➤ Place two fingers on the carotid artery in the neck (pic. 1) or the inner wrist (pic. 2).

➤ Count the total number of beats for 30 seconds then double the number – this is your resting heart rate.

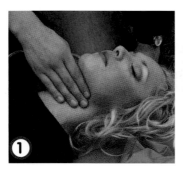
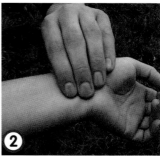

The average is around 75 beats to the minute. Slightly lower is excellent, but if your count is 85 or higher then you could have a problem. Bear in mind, however, that pain and anxiety can produce a faster-than-normal pulse rate in a casualty.

Taking Body Temperature

Take a clinical thermometer, holding it with your thumb and fingers by the top end of the scale (opposite to the bulb end) and flick your wrist two or three times to cancel the previous reading. Place the thermometer under the casualty's tongue and leave in place for about three minutes (longer if in very cold conditions). Remove and record the temperature from the scale. The armpit, groin and rectum may also be used for taking temperature.

The chart opposite shows normal body temperatures.

NORMAL BODY TEMPERATURES

Mouth	97–99°F	36–37°C
Armpit	97–99°F	36–37°C
Groin	97–99°F	36–37°C
Rectum	98–100°F	36.5–38°C

Wounds

BLOOD LOSS

It is vital that severe blood loss is stemmed as soon as possible. The body reacts to any wound by contracting the blood vessels in the immediate area. As blood exits the wound it solidifies and forms into a blood clot that effectively seals the wound. Almost immediately the body's defence mechanisms will start to repair the damage and combat any infection. How well this works will depend on the amount of damage and the severity of the wound. Where blood loss is severe, the body will shut down

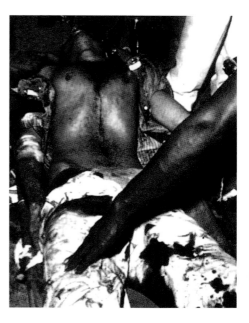

Stemming blood loss is the priority after stabilising breathing and circulation

most of the peripheral blood vessels thus maintaining a good supply of blood to the vital organs.

Types of Bleeding

Once the type of wound is established check for the type of bleeding.

➤ **Blood from a ruptured artery** will normally be bright red in colour and propel itself from the wound in short spurts in time with the heartbeat.

➤ **Blood from a vein** will extrude at a lower pressure and be darker in colour.

More often than not blood loss looks worse than it really is and patients should be assured of this. However, severe arterial bleeding must be treated immediately as this can induce shock.

Types of Wound

Simple graze

The most common type of blood loss is from a simple graze which results when skin is scraped against a rough surface, for example, due to a fall on rocky ground. Although not normally deep a simple graze can harbour a lot of dirt and fragmentation which becomes embedded in the wound.

Contused wound

A more serious wound can be caused by fall or when a blow has been delivered to the body by a blunt object. This is termed as a contused wound which has a tendency to split the skin rather than cut it. Serious contused wounds are normally accompanied by bruising around the damaged skin, indicating that there may be damage behind the wound.

Ragged cuts

Cuts with a ragged edge caused by broken glass, wire or an animal attack leave a lacerated wound. Due to the ragged edge the wound will produce good clotting and thus limit the amount of bleeding.

Incised wounds

An incised wound is normally a clean cut caused by a knife or razor edged tool or weapon. The wound will bleed a lot due to the fact that the blood vessels are clean-cut and do not contract easily.

Puncture wounds

A puncture wound is caused when a pointed object such as a nail enters the body. Deep puncture wounds can be serious as they carry the risk of infection which cannot be treated in the same way as an open wound.

BLOOD FROM AN ORIFICE

➤ If the victim is vomiting dark red blood it could indicate an injury to the digestive system.

➤ Coughed-up bright red frothy blood could indicate damage to the upper airways or lungs, possibly caused by a fractured rib.

➤ Sticky straw-coloured blood from the ear could indicate a fractured skull.

(Cont'd)

> ➤ Stools which contain black tarry blood indicates bleeding from the upper intestine.

> ➤ Blood stained urine could indicate kidney or bladder damage.

Controlling Severe Blood Loss

WARNING

> ➤ Do not let severe blood loss distract you from observing the proper priorities of treatment. Perform the ABC regime (see p.22) then attend to the bleeding.

A wound which causes a deep or large incision in the body, or an accidental amputation of a limb, will produce serious blood loss. Most external wounds with excessive bleeding are highly visual and require immediate attention. You should make sure the casualty is placed in the most suitable position for treatment and always examine the wound to check for the presence of any foreign material before applying any treatment. There are three main options open to the medic for controlling blood loss: direct pressure, indirect pressure and elevation.

Direct Pressure

Place a dressing over the wound and apply firm but gentle pressure with the hand. A sterile dressing is preferable, but if one is not available, any piece of clean cloth can be used (see pic. 1).

If there is nothing immediately available, cover the wound with your hand. If necessary, hold the edges of the wound together with gentle pressure (pics 2, 3). Any dressings used should be large enough to overlap the wound and cover the surrounding area. If blood comes through the first dressing, apply a second over the first, and a third over the second if required. Keep even pressure applied by tying on a firm bandage. Take great care that the bandage is not so tight that, like a tourniquet, it restricts the flow of blood.

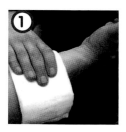
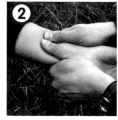
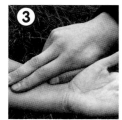

If the wound is large and suitable dressings are to hand, bring the edges of the wound together and use the dressings to keep the wound closed. To arrest the flow of blood from a very large wound, make a pad of the dressing and press it in to the wound where the bleeding is heaviest.

The object of this treatment is to slow down or stop the loss of blood until the body's own defences come into play. The blood will clot relatively quickly if the flow is slowed or stopped. Although a cleanly cut blood vessel may bleed profusely, it will shrink, close and retreat into its surrounding tissue if left untreated. Sometimes these natural processes will succeed in arresting bleeding entirely unaided. Reassurance and rest play a vital part in the treatment because they can lower the rate of heartbeat and so reduce the flowrate of blood around the body.

Elevation

If there is no danger of any other injury being aggravated, an injured limb is best raised as high as is comfortable for the casualty. This reduces the blood flow to the limb, helps the veins to drain the area and so assists in reducing the blood loss through the wound.

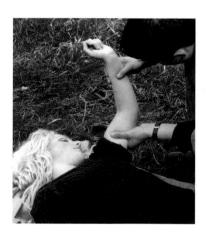

Indirect Pressure

If a combination of these procedures does not succeed, the use of appropriate pressure points must be considered. First, it is necessary to recognise the type of external bleeding (see p.57), because pressure points can only be used to control arterial bleeding.

A place where an artery runs across a bone near the surface of the skin constitutes a pressure point. There

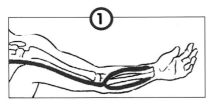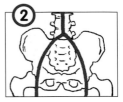

The brachial arteries (pic. 1) and the femoral artieries (pic. 2)

are four pressure points readily available to control heavy arterial bleeding – one in each limb. Those in the arms are on the brachial arteries which run down the centre of the inner side of the upper arm (pic. 1).

Pressure points for the legs are on the femoral arteries, which run down the inside of the thigh (pic. 2). The pressure points can be found in the centre of the groin, and can be compressed against the pelvis. This is easier to do if the casualty's knee is bent. When using pressure points to control bleeding make full use of the opportunity to dress the wound more effectively.

PRESSURE APPLICATION

➤ Locate the fingers or thumb over the pressure point and apply sufficient pressure to flatten the artery and arrest the flow of blood.

➤ Redress the wound.

➤ Maintain the pressure for at least ten minutes to allow time for blood-clotting to begin. **DO NOT EXCEED 15 MINUTES** or the tissues below the pressure point will begin to be damaged by the deprivation of arterial blood. It is essential to release the controlling pressure after **15 MINUTES**.

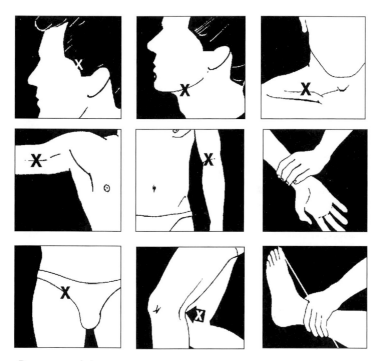

Pressure points

Tourniquet

If the damage to a limb is so severe it plainly requires amputation, or if part of the limb is missing, and direct pressure will not stop the bleeding, you may need to apply a tourniquet. The tourniquet can be made from whatever cloth is at hand, but avoid using any thin material that will cut into the flesh.

➤   Place it around the extremity, between the wound and the heart, 5–10 centimetres (2–4 inches) above the wound site (pic. 1, p. 64). Never place it directly over the wound or a fracture.

➤ Use a stick as a handle to tighten the tourniquet and tighten it only enough to stop blood flow (pics. 2, 3).

➤ Clean and bandage the wound.

➤ The tourniquet must be slowly released every 10–15 minutes for a period of 1–2 minutes, but you must continue to apply direct pressure at all times.

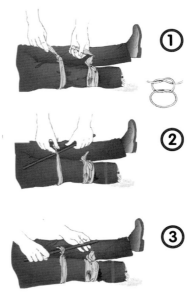

WARNING

➤ Applying a tourniquet to prevent blood flow is a dangerous procedure and should only be attempted when all else has failed.

Self-Help

It is possible that you may become injured while you are on your own, in which case it is sensible to have thought out a self-help routine:

➤ Try to rest. Lie down somewhere, but preferably out of the wind.

➤ Use direct pressure on your wound to control the bleeding. Apply a dressing, sterile or improvised, if possible.

➤ Tie it firmly but not so tight as to restrict circulation.

➤ If possible, elevate the injury and support it. Pain will be less if you try and keep as still as possible. Try and make sure that you can keep warm.

➤ You may have to be prepared to lose a limb to save your life.

INTERNAL BLEEDING

Internal bleeding is a serious condition that requires immediate medical attention. The cause of internal bleeding varies depending on the history. The more common causes are from a crush injury, deep penetrating wound, such as a missile, which has damaged a major organ, or a stomach ulcer.

Not all internal bleeding is self-evident and there may be no external signs to indicate blood loss. Although the blood remains in the body it is lost from the circulation, starving the vital organs of oxygen. In certain areas, this build-up of blood can cause additional problems. For example, internal bleeding in the skull can put pressure on the brain, and in the chest it can prevent the lungs from expanding.

Always suspect internal bleeding if the casualty has been involved in a violent injury. Internal bleeding is difficult to detect and treat, however, it is possible to get some indication by performing a capillary refill test.

Capilliary Refill Test

Depress one of the casualty's fingernails or the tip of a finger for 5 seconds (I find the pad of the thumb best) and note the white to pink reaction. In a normal response the capillary bed will regain its colour within two seconds. A slower rate of colour return may indicate internal blood loss. Check the casualty for any obvious crush injury, loss of blood into the chest, abdomen or pelvis and thigh are all possibilities.

Look for the following signs of internal bleeding.

INTERNAL BLEEDING INDICATORS

➤ Evidence of a severe blow or violent crush injury

➤ Pain, bruising or swelling

➤ A pale, cold, clammy skin

➤ A rapid and weak pulse

➤ Restlessness and thirst

➤ Tenderness over the abdomen

➤ Signs of shock

TREATMENT

➤ If injuries allow, lay the casualty down and elevate the legs in order to facilitate blood to the vital organs

➤ If the casualty is conscious, place them in the position most comfortable for them.

➤ Loosen any restrictive clothing.

➤ Minimise shock (see p.68) and look for other injuries.

➤ If the casualty is dehydrated, water can be given.

The scope of this book prevents any further treatment for acute internal bleeding other than to watch for signs of shock. In the case of internal bleeding as the condition becomes more acute it is accompanied by a rising pulse rate. Where serious internal bleeding is suspected immediate evacuation should be organized.

AUTHOR'S NOTE

➤ I have seen several men shot, and all received prompt and expert treatment from the patrol medic. However, on at least two occasions the casualties have died from internal bleeding. Both men were conscious and apart from the injury pain they proclaimed to feel fine. The hidden internal bleeding had gone undetected both by the medic and the casualties.

SHOCK

Shock is a condition resulting from either illness or injury, which reduces the volume of blood or fluid, causing weakness to the body. Often referred to as traumatic or injury shock, it is a serious condition which can be fatal, even after bodily injuries have been treated. In the initial stages, the condition is reversible, but if shock is prolonged it will become irreversible and result in death.

CAUSES OF SHOCK

➤ Blood loss from either external or internal bleeding

➤ Loss of plasma from severe burns

➤ Heart attack

➤ Severe abdominal emergencies

➤ Loss of water from intestinal blockage

➤ Recurrent vomiting

➤ Severe diarrhoea

➤ Extreme cases of pain or fear can also produce shock symptoms

Causes

There are a number of reasons why a casualty can go into shock but the common cause in all cases is inadequate capillary perfusion. This book does not have the capacity to deal with all forms of shock and is restricted to the diagnosis and treatment of shock developing from acute blood loss as this is by far the most commonly encountered shock syndrome.

SYMPTOMS OF SHOCK

➤ The person will be weak, feel faint, and at the same time restless and anxious.

➤ There may be a feeling of sickness or a need to vomit.

➤ The person may be thirsty.

➤ The skin becomes cold, clammy and pale, with possible sweating.

➤ The person may yawn or sigh, with shallow, rapid breathing.

➤ The person may yawn or sigh, with shallow, rapid breathing.

➤ The pulse will increase but also become weaker and sometimes irregular, due to blood and fluid loss.

➤ There will be decreased blood flow to the skin.

➤ Unconsciousness may develop.

TREATMENT

Treatment for shock should be based on rest, reassurance and dealing with the underlying cause of the shock.

➤ If injuries allow, lay the casualty down with the head slightly lower than the body. Providing there are no leg injuries these can be raised slightly to help maintain the blood supply to the heart lungs and brain.

➤ If no spinal injuries are suspected, turn the head to one side to lessen the dangers of vomiting and possible asphyxia.

➤ Loosen any restrictive clothing and cover the casualty to keep them warm. Be careful not to cause overheating (e.g. by adding a water bottle) as this will increase the blood supply to the skin surface thus robbing the vital organs.

➤ Monitor breathing, pulse and responsiveness every 10 minutes.

WOUND INFECTION

Open wounds of any kind, however small, risk contamination and the development of infection. The amount of infection is directly related to the amount of time between wounding and treatment. The longer the delay the more time the bacteria have to multiply. Early treatment prevents the infection becoming established, thus prompt and adequate treatment is crucial in avoiding wound infection. Delays can lead to poor wound healing and even death. A course of suitable antibiotics will help control the infection. One or more of the following factors governs the main cause of wound infection.

Causes of Wound Infection

➤ Delay in treatment

➤ Inadequate cleaning of the wound

➤ Foreign bodies left within the wound

➤ Inadequate drainage

➤ Non-sterile dressing

SIGNS OF WOUND INFECTION

➤ Pain and tenderness

➤ Swelling

➤ Redness spreading from the edges of the wound

➤ Heat around the affected area

➤ Fever may set in if the infection is not controlled

➤ Rigors and chills may indicate a resulting blood poisoning

TETANUS

In both developed and developing countries, especially those with warmer climates, tetanus can be a real risk. Tetanus may develop where wounds are left to become infected with the *Clostridium tetani* bacterium. This toxin causes muscle contractions and spasms leading to exhaustion and a failed respiratory system. Once the tetanus toxin has established itself in the body and in the absence of specialised treatment, death is likely to occur. The first signs of the disease are normally detected when the jaw muscles go into spasm.

TREATMENT

The best prevention is immunisation. Where a person has never received a tetanus shot (or a booster in the preceding 10 years) and medical aid is not forthcoming, the best solution is to keep the wound clean (see below). Deep wounds resulting from a contaminated source (such as an animal bite) or those wounds that have been subject to immersion in dirty water are particularly vulnerable and must be closely watched.

WOUND CLEANING

The purpose of washing a wound is to remove as much bacteria as possible, and so give the body's defensive system the best chance of finishing the job. All exposed wounds, no matter how small, need to be kept clean. This is best done with water that has been sterilised by boiling, but clean, pure drinking water will suffice if boiling is not possible (in emergencies, male urine can be used). Deeper wounds can be washed out more efficiently by using an irrigation bulb which will provide a strong jet of water into the wound. If you do not have one, then improvise with a small plastic bottle or polythene bag into which a small pin-sized hole has been made, allowing the water to be squeezed out. Adding antibacterial soap to the water (the mixture should be sufficiently weak as to scarcely cloud one pint of water) will help to thoroughly clean the wound. If this is not available, consider dissolving a small amount of potassium permanganate crystals into water: you should use barely enough to colour a pint of water. If you are unsure as to the correct concentrations, err on the side of caution and keep it very dilute – drinking a small amount without any ill effects is a good test of the right strength.

Procedure

➤ Before beginning, open the wound to its fullest extent and examine for foreign debris, such as bits of clothing or glass, or any material that may have been forced into the wound.

➤ If no proper sterile instruments are available, wash your hands with soap and water and use your fingers.

➤ Once the wound is open, scrub briskly, irrigating at the same time; a job best done with two people.

➤ Work quickly as this will prove very painful for the patient.

➤ Once finished apply a clean sterile dressing and arrest any fresh bleeding by direct pressure. Check the wound on a daily basis.

WARNING

➤ In many isolated regions of the world local peoples have devised their own form of wound healing. Such wound treatments as the ancient Arabic tradition of burning wounds with a hot iron, or the theatrical methods of pouring gun powder into a wound and setting fire to it may work, but the risk of creating a wound larger than the original is very high. Such methods only serve to kill both live and dead tissue.

WOUND CLOSURE

In general, wounds older than 6–8 hours should not be closed. In the wilderness, wound closure should be limited to the use of butterfly closures. These are similar to plasters, in

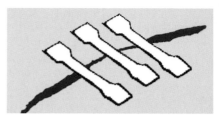

Butterfly sutures

as much that they have a sticky surface which adheres to the skin and can be used to hold together small to medium-sized, straight-edged cuts. In an emergency, duct tape or similar can be used as an alternative.

Procedure

➤ Ensure the area surrounding the wound is clean and completely dry before applying the butterflies

➤ Pinch the edges together and tape across the length of the wound at 0.5 cm ($^1/_4$ inch) intervals

➤ Secure the ends of the butterflies by taping over them with longer strips of plaster running parallel to the wound

➤ Cover the wound with a clean and preferably sterile, non-stick dressing

➤ Check dressings every 24 hours for infection (see p.70) and change every 24–48 hours or when wet or dirty

Bandaging of Wounds

There is a wide range of wound dressings and many ways of applying them, but most are simple and straightforward. Where a manufactured dressing is not available use some kind of clean, non-fluffy material such as clothing, bedding or towels. Whatever you use the dressing should be large enough to cover and overlap the wound. The principle of a direct dressing is to control bleeding, protect the wound from infection and to absorb fluid from the wound.

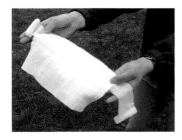 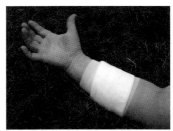

Dressings may also be used to facilitate splints, or hold a limb in a specified position.

Sucking Chest Wounds

If air is allowed to enter the lungs from puncture wounds to the chest or back, then a sucking wound will develop. Always check for sucking wounds if missiles of any form have penetrated deeply, or a rib is protruding from the chest or back. The lung on the affected side will collapse and as the casualty breathes in, the sucked air will also impair the effi-

SUCKING CHEST WOUND SYMPTOMS

➤ Chest pain
➤ The sound of air being sucked in from the chest
➤ Difficulty in breathing
➤ Bright blood bubbling from a chest wound
➤ Blueness around the mouth

ciency of the good lung if the condition goes untreated. The result is a lack of oxygen reaching the bloodstream that could cause asphyxia.

TREATMENT

If a sucking wound is suspected:

➤ Immediately cover the area with your hand.

➤ Support the casualty in a lop-sided sitting position
with the functioning lung down.

➤ Cover the wound with a clean dressing and place
a plastic sheet over the top so that the plastic
overlaps the dressing and wound. Tape down to
form an airtight seal (pics. 1 and 2).

➤ Leave one of the lower corners free so that air
can escape when the casualty exhales.

➤ Place the casualty's arm on the injured side
across their chest and support it with a
triangular sling (pic. 3)

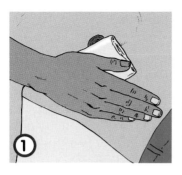

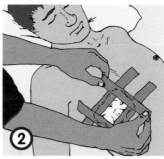

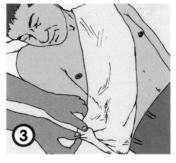

➤ If a foreign body is present in the wound, do not remove, but pack with a ring dressing and fit an airtight seal, leaving one side free.

➤ Arrange to have the casualty evacuated as soon as possible.

ABDOMINAL WOUNDS

Injuries of the abdomen may be

➤ **closed,** that is, with no external wound present, or

➤ **open** with a wound through the abdominal wall.

Open wounds are more commonly seen where some form of impalement or missile injury has taken place.

Closed abdominal wounds are normally caused by blows over the abdominal wall, but they can also be caused by blast. An injury like this produces no wound on the skin surface but may damage the internal organs. The damage may be to solid organs such as the liver, spleen or kidneys, or to hollow organs like the intestinal tract, or both.

In general, damage to solid organs produces internal bleeding, when the bleeding is not visible the blood may collect within the abdominal cavity. Damage to hollow organs also causes some bleeding although usually not so severe, but it also allows the contents of the organ to spill out into the abdominal cavity. In the bowel these contents are highly irritant to the peritoneal lining and give rise to serious infection.

TREATMENT

There is little that can be done for a serious penetration of the abdominal cavity, especially if the wound is caused by a missile, but the following steps should be taken:

➤ Carry out the ABC regime (see p.22) if necessary

➤ Lay the casualty down and raise their knees. This will minimise any muscle and skin stretching of the abdominal wall.

➤ Control any external bleeding (see p.59)

➤ Clean the entry wound and apply a moist dressing (see p.72)

➤   Check for signs of internal bleeding (see p.65)

➤   Check for and treat any shock (see p.68)

The bleeding can only be stopped by operation and the patient may also need a blood transfusion. They should be evacuated to a medical facility as soon as possible.

GUNSHOT & MISSILE WOUNDS

All guns are dangerous, and can cause horrific damage to the human body. Wounds can range from minor, superficial skin wounds to major organ injury causing instant death. The degree of wounding will vary depending on the type of weapon and the location of the injury. Low velocity projectiles such as those fired from a shotgun may penetrate and remain in the body, while high velocity bullets fired from a military-type weapon will almost certainly make an entry and an exit wound. The track of the missile also makes a difference, for if the bullet hits bone it can splinter and be deflected. High velocity bullets also emit energy in the form of shock waves which are powerful enough to severely damage flesh along the missile track. The angle of the bullet as it impacts with the body can also make a difference. If it is travelling normally then it will enter the body in a straight line. If, however, the bullet has yawed or spun as it travels and enters the body sideways on, the damage will be greatly increased. The composition of the bullet, be it hard or soft, will also make a large difference.

TREATMENT

➤ Perform the ABC regime (see p.22)

➤ Control the bleeding (see p.59)

➤ Treat the casualty for shock (see p.68)

➤ Monitor the breathing and pulse continually.

➤ Remove any debris from both entry and exit wounds and extensively irrigate and clean (see Wound Cleaning, p.72).

➤ Dress with a sterile bandage and administer antibiotics, if available

Keen observation to ascertain the missile entry point, and if perforating, the exit point, should help establish the missile track. If the missile has entered the torso the position should give a good indication of possible organ damage. For example, a wound to the right side of the chest would indicate lung damage. With missile wounds to the limbs you should first look for bone fracture. In all cases check for damage to the major blood vessels.

EXCESSIVE NOSE BLEEDS

Bleeding from the nose is a common symptom and may be due to local or general causes. However, in some cases continual nose bleeding can cause asphyxia. Excessive nose bleeding can be caused by:

➤ Injury to the nose

➤ Fracture of the base of the skull

➤ Ulceration of the nasal mucus membrane

➤ High blood pressure

➤ Mountain sickness

➤ Blood diseases such as leukaemia

➤ Typhoid fever

TREATMENT

➤ The patient should sit erect and the clothing around the neck loosened while breathing through an opened mouth.

➤ A cold compress or ice bag may be applied to the nose. (Wet a cloth and waft it through the air to cool it.)

➤ Pinching the soft parts of the nose gently for five minutes may be sufficient to stop the bleeding.

➤ No attempt to blow the nose or sneeze should be made for the next 48 hours.

➤ If these methods fail, and removal to a medical facility is not possible, the affected side must be plugged lightly with ribbon gauze. The plugging must be removed after 12 hours to prevent it becoming septic.

FOREIGN BODIES

In the wilderness, foreign bodies can include gravel, wood splinters or even insects. Smaller fragments and projectiles like broken glass can be removed (but **not** from the eyes).

Unless life-threatening, larger foreign bodies which are embedded should be left in place because pulling at them may do further damage. Instead, control the bleeding by direct pressure, squeezing the wound in line with the foreign body. Next form a padded ring which will fit neatly over the protruding object and secure it with a dressing.

Objects in the Eye

SAFETY RULES FOR EYE INJURIES

➤ Under no circumstances should an untrained or inexperienced person attempt to remove a foreign body embedded in the eyeball.

➤ Immediately after an injury, the eye may be bathed with a suitable antiseptic.

➤ The eye should be covered with a sterile bandage.

➤ The casualty should be evacuated immediately.

Dislocations & Fractures

DISLOCATIONS

Dislocations are caused when bone joints (particularly of the shoulders, elbows, hips, fingers or knees) become separated and move out of alignment. This can be extremely painful as the nerve and blood flow are affected.

DISLOCATION SYMPTOMS

➤ Deformity (the injured limb will seem distorted compared to an uninjured one)

➤ Severe pain

➤ Inability to move the damaged part

The management of dislocated limbs is very similar to that of fractures to the same body part (see p. 85). However, if blood flow to the injured limb is impaired or there is a lengthy delay in getting the casualty to professional medical help, then the best way to relieve this painful condition is to realign the joint as quickly as possible.

There are two basic methods, depending on whether the casualty is alone or not.

Treating When Alone

The lone casualty will need to improvise some form of weight, a large rock or log, to which they can attach a cord from the limb. The idea is to stretch the limb slightly by countering against the weight and aligning back into place. The procedure requires the body and or limb to be rotated in order to set the joint while at the same time comparing it to the joint on the opposite side. All movement must be kept to a minimum, yet be positive. The procedure should be done lying down as it is extremely painful and the manoeuvre will require a great deal of will-power.

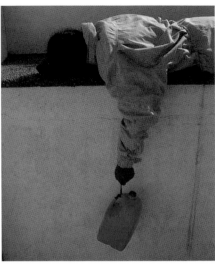

Treating When Assisted

The same basic procedure of stretching and realigning the limb as above, but it is far more likely to be successful. Where possible one person should hold the casualty in a comfortable position while a second manipulates the limb into alignment. Again this procedure is best done with the casualty lying down

Both, if successful, will bring about a lowering of pain and restoration of blood circulation. Once completed the limb should be immobilized using splints if possible and allowed to recover. Use a well-padded splint above and below the fracture site. Always check the circulation below the dislocation after completing the splint. Remove the splint after a week and start gentle exercises until the limb is fully functional.

FRACTURES

In a wilderness situation, the scope for treatment of a fracture is limited to immobilisation of the injured part. Splints should be applied before the casualty is moved unless there is imminent danger which requires immediate evacuation. If conscious, the casualty will be experiencing pain, so handle them with the greatest of care so as not to cause increased distress. If the fracture has also caused a wound, this must be treated and stabilised (see p. 56) before any splints are fitted.

FRACTURE SYMPTOMS

➤ Difficulty in normal movement of any part of the body
➤ Increased pain when movement is attempted
➤ Swelling or bruising accompanied by tenderness in the area of the injury
➤ Deformity or shortening of the injured part

(Cont'd)

➤ Grating of bone heard during examination or attempted movement

➤ Signs of shock

➤ The injured having heard or felt a bone break

Types of Fracture

Simple

The bone is completely broken and the surrounding tissue is damaged (either completely or partially torn). In a simple fracture the bones are free to move around, and as the ends of the bone are very sharp, they can do considerable damage to surrounding muscle; because of this, considerable blood loss around the area of the fracture is common. This can cause the casualty will go into shock (see p. 68), becoming pale, cold and sweating, with a rapid pulse rate of around 100 beats per minute. The muscle around the fracture will still be working, pulling the fragments in different directions. Sometimes they cause the broken ends to overlap, which in the leg or thigh, where this type of fracture is common, can shorten the leg by several inches.

Compound

This is a more complicated fracture to treat because it is a fracture that is exposed to air. Consequently, there is a greater chance of infection which can delay

Compound fracture

the healing process and if severe enough, result in the loss of the limb or even death.

Complicated

A complicated fracture involves damage to blood vessels or and this can have serious and permanent effects. For example, if a nerve is cut all feeling is lost in the limb below this level and muscles which are supplied by the nerve can become paralysed. Even though a nerve can be repaired it can take up to two years to reach the end of the limb.

Comminuted

This is when the bone is broken into several pieces, which means that it will be very weak and unstable. It takes a considerable force to create this kind of fracture.

Treating Fractures

Skull Fractures and Concussion

All head injuries must be regarded as serious, even if a head wound looks slight. A direct blow to the head or a fall can cause a fracture to the cranium (the crown of the head) but damage to the skull bone may not necessarily be evident. For example, there may be a depressed fracture or an internal leakage of blood from a fracture which could cause pressure to the

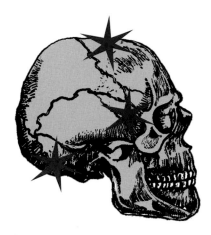

Common fracture sites of the skull

brain itself. Also, a blow to the jaw or an indirect force, such as landing hard on your feet from a high jump, can cause a fracture to the base of the skull. Concussion is a temporary disturbance of the brain normally due to a severe blow or shaking.

A skull fracture or concussion must be suspected if any or all of the following symptoms are present.

SKULL FRACTURE SYMPTOMS

➤ An obvious head wound, bruise or a soft or depressed area on the scalp

➤ Unconsciousness, even for a short period of time

➤ Clear fluid or watery blood coming from the ears or nose

➤ Blood in the white of the eye

➤ The pupils of the eyes are unequal or unresponsive

➤ A steady deterioration in responsiveness to external stimuli

TREATMENT

If conscious, the casualty should be made to lie down with their head and shoulders supported. If unconscious, perform the ABC regime immediately (see p. 22). If the casualty is unconscious but breathing and pulse are normal, place them in the recovery position (see p. 29) and maintain a close check on their vital signs. In either case, make sure that the casualty is kept warm and quiet and handled carefully. Apply a light padding to the injured area and hold it in place with dressing. If blood is being discharged from an ear, lightly cover, but do not block. Concussion is normally only a temporary disturbance from which the chances of recovery are good.

Limb Fractures

The majority of fractures are limb fractures. While fractures to the arms are incapacitating and will require medical treatment in a hospital, leg fractures usually cause immobility and therefore require an evacuation. The first priority, providing the airway is not affected – if it is, see p. 22 – is to determine the extent of the injury and control any bleeding (see p. 59).

LIMB FRACTURE SYMPTOMS

➤ Deformity
➤ Exposed bone
➤ Swelling and discolouration

(Cont'd)

➤ Pain at the fracture site which is worsened by any movement

➤ Loss of movement to the limb

TREATMENT

The only treatment available in an emergency situation is to clean and dress any wound (if required, see p.72), splint the fracture and immobilise the limb. Treat for shock (see p.68). Unless some other immediate danger threatens, splint the casualty before moving them. In any case, handle with the greatest care to avoid further pain or additional injury.

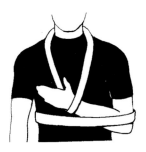

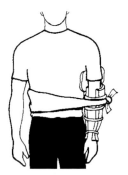

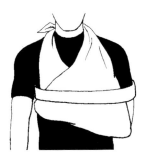

Immobilising a fractured arm: further support for a fractured arm can be achieved by binding the injured limb to the body using a broad bandage to restrict its movement

SPLINTING

Good splinting helps prevent further damage to the tissues surrounding a fracture while the casualty is being transported and also reduces bleeding and pain. Manufactured splints (carried in medical packs) come in a wide variety of shapes and materials, although in an emergency, suitable splints can be improvised from small branches, sticks and suitable pieces of equipment, rolled clothing or bedding. 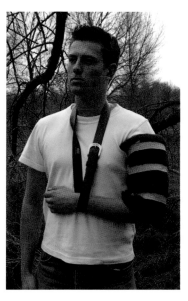 Make sure any splint is padded and that it supports the joints both above and below the fracture. In the case of a leg fracture, if no suitable substitute for a splint can be found in your environment, immobilise it by tying it to the good leg instead.

WARNING

➤ Do not tie splints directly over an injury or allow knots supporting a sling to press against an injury.

Use gentle traction to realign the limb, providing the casualty can tolerate the pain. Pull gently in a straight line with the bone until the limb has been straightened. Done properly, the casualty may find that the pain and any bleeding at the site of the fracture are significantly reduced. Once you have done all you can to straighten the limb, apply the splints. If possible, elevate and support the fractured limb as this will help to reduce any swelling or any chance of the casualty going into shock. Make sure that the casualty receives plenty of rest. Once the splint has been applied, test for the capilliary refill time (see p.66). If this is greater than 2 seconds, re-apply the splint and fasten in a slightly loosewr fashion.

WARNING

➤ Check periodically that the casualty's circulation is not being impeded by any splint or bandage. Blue or ashen fingers or toes are an obvious indicator that the bindings are too tight.

Arms and Wrist Fractures

Fractures to this part of the body often result from a person trying to protect themselves by using their arms or hands to break a fall, or from striking a hard object during a fall. Fractures in these areas are often accompanied by severe pain when moving the affected part, with swelling and deformity at the site.

TREATMENT

For a fracture to the arm Place the forearm gently across the casualty's chest while supporting it (pic. 1). Place padding between the arm and the chest and use a sling to support the arm (pic. 2). Alternatively, use a strap looped around the wrist and neck to allow the arm to hang as if in a sling, which may be more comfortable (pic. 3). Strap the upper arm to the body with a broad bandage to provide complete immobilisation. A rigid splint on the affected part of the arm may also be used.

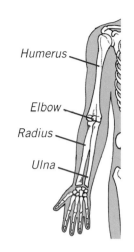

Humerus

Elbow

Radius

Ulna

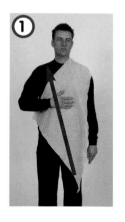

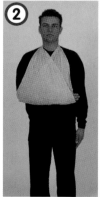

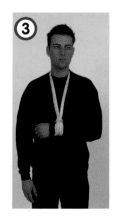

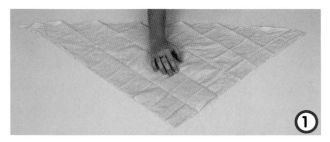

For a fracture to the wrist
Check the wrist pulse (without moving the hand) to ensure that the injury is not restricting blood supply to the hand. Pad the hand and wrist to provide additional

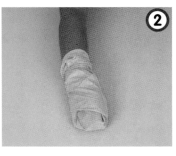

protection (pics 1, 2) before applying a sling and positioning it so that the hand is elevated above the elbow (pic. 3). Strap the affected arm to the body for complete immobilisation (pic. 4).

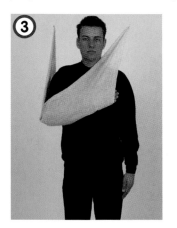

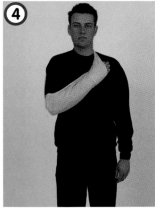

Rib Fractures

A direct blow or an object falling on the chest normally causes rib fractures. Depending on the amount of force and the

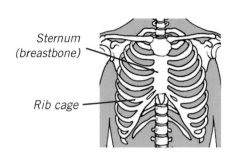

Sternum (breastbone)

Rib cage

angle of the blow, rib fractures can be complicated by a sucking wound (see p. 75) or if the chest is stove in, breathing can be impeded.

BROKEN RIB SYMPTOMS

➤ Sharp pain at the site of the fracture
➤ Difficulty in breathing
➤ Open chest wound
➤ Bruising under the skin

TREATMENT

Treatment should be based on the ABC regime (see p. 22) and immobilising the fracture. Lay the casualty down in a relaxed sitting position with the head and shoulders supported and the body leaning towards the injured side. Place a pad over any exposed wound and hold this in place by placing the casualty's (injured side) arm in a sling (see p. 93). If a rib bone is exposed through the chest wall it is likely that the lung will also be damaged (see Sucking Wounds, p. 75).

Hip or Thigh Fractures

A broken thigh or hip can be caused by either a fall or a mid- to lower body crush injury. Check the injured area for swelling, redness or bruising. Next carefully remove or open any footwear and feel for a pulse on the top of the foot. If no pulse is detected, it could indicate that the main arteries have been damaged.

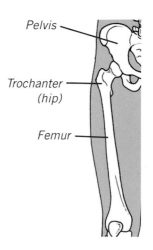

Pelvis

Trochanter (hip)

Femur

TREATMENT

Gently straighten the injured leg, making sure the traction is in line with the leg's normal position. Place some form of padding between the legs and fix a splint

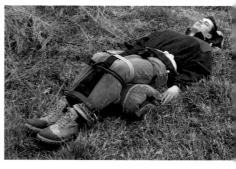

down the whole length of the injured leg. Next secure both legs together by applying straps above and below the knees and around the ankles.

Although internal bleeding may be present there is little that can be done until the casualty reaches hospital. Concentrate your efforts on preventing shock (see p. 68).

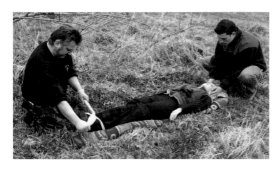

Straps applied above and below the knees and around the ankles secure both legs.

Lower Leg Fractures

Fractures of the lower leg are often obvious, with the leg or foot resting at an abnormal angle, accompanied by severe pain and swelling and an inability to bear any weight on the affected leg; fractures of the tibia may also break the skin (see Complicated Fractures, p. 87). A broken fibula may only cause pain on the outer side of the leg alone. A fracture or dislocation of the kneecap may have tenderness on the inner side of the knee, swelling and (possibly severe) pain when attempting to straighten the knee.

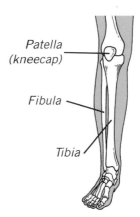

Patella (kneecap)

Fibula

Tibia

TREATMENT

The casualty should be lying down. Treat any wounds (see p. 56) and for shock (see p. 68) as necessary. Gently straighten the leg with traction at the ankle. Splint the affected limb from above the knee to below the heel. Alternatively, if no splints are available, pad between the knees and tie the legs together.

For a kneecap fracture, place a splint behind the leg running from buttock to heel and pad the natural hollows under the knee and ankle and bind at the thigh, shin and ankle.

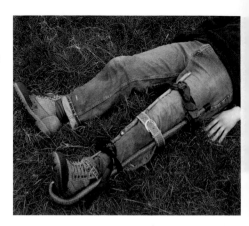

Foot Injury

Foot and ankle injuries are a serious concern when backpacking in the wilderness as they limit mobility. In many cases the injury will have occurred as a result of a twisting fall on hard ground.

TREATMENT

Rest the casualty and decide whether to remove the boot or not. Be aware that if you take the boot off, depending on the injury, you may not be able to get it

---

FOOT INJURY SYMPTOMS

➤ Pain which is increased by movement
➤ Tenderness to the touch.
➤ Bruising and swelling.

(Cont'd)

➤ Deformity.

➤ If the casualty can walk a few (albeit painful) steps, then an ankle injury may only be a sprain. Being unable to do this however, does not automatically indicate a fracture as a severe sprain may not allow the casualty to put weight on the affected foot.

back on. It is best to leave the boot on if:

➤ you plan to walk out

➤ the weather is bad or deteriorating

➤ the terrain is difficult.

If you do remove the footwear and stocking from the damaged foot, place a thick pad under the base of the foot and secure with a criss-cross bandage that reaches up around and supports the ankle.

Improvised foot splints

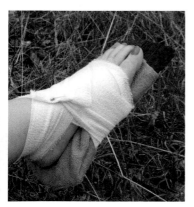 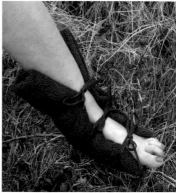

Back or Spine Injury

If a person has fallen from a height or they have been
knocked over by a vehicle, there is always the prospect
of back injury (and possibly a head injury, see p.87 for
assessment and treatment).

WARNING

➤ Unless the casualty's life is in immediate danger do not move
them. While the casualty may not have any apparent injury,
moving them may result in spinal cord damage. Similarly, do
not bend or twist the casualty's head, neck or back during
any examination

In a wilderness situation where help may be slow in
coming, you will need to assess the degree of possible
damage to the spine. However, if the casualty is
unconscious, perform the ABC regime (see p.22)
immediately and place in the spinal recovery position
described below if possible.

SPINAL RECOVERY POSITION

➤ Six people are required. One person positions
themself at the casualty's head and is responsible
for ensuring the head, neck and spine remain in
a straight line during any movement. This
person gives the orders to the others for any
move (pic. 1).

➤ Three people kneel on one side of the casualty
and two on the other (pic. 1).

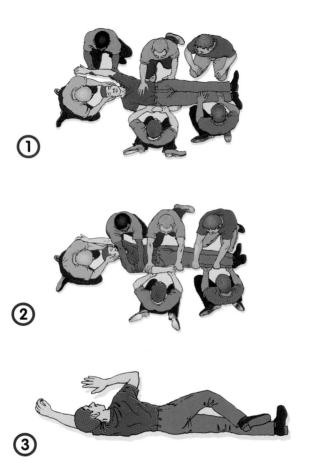

➤ One of the casualty's arms should be positioned straight up beside his head and the three helpers must carefully roll him onto the side with the raised arm, avoiding any twisting of his back as they do so. The two helpers must carefully provide support and lift as the casualty rolls over (pic. 2).

➤ The casualty's head should rest on the raised arm to keep the line of the neck and spine straight.

➤ Bend the upper leg so that knee and calf rest across the lower leg with the head neck and body in alignment (pic. 3).

➤ Support the body on both sides if necessary to maintain this position

If the casualty is conscious, ensure they do not move. Begin your assessment by asking them what happened, where any impact points were and where it hurts. Then touch the casualty's fingers, arms, and toes to check for sensitivity and ask the casualty to move these parts each in turn. Loss of movement and feeling in any of these areas could indicate an injury to the spinal cord.

The following signs may also be present:

➤ Pain and deformity

➤ Paralysis

➤ Loss of bladder/bowel control

➤ Muscle spasm

➤ A tingling sensation below an obvious injury point.

TREATMENT

There is little that can be done for severe back injuries other than to evacuate to a medical facility as soon as possible. To immobilise the casualty:

➤ One person should support either side of the head (using a knee on either side of the head is easier on the helper's back than prolonged

bending over)

➤ Support the body with solid objects (e.g. logs)

➤ Place soft padding between the legs and bind them together at the hips, thighs and ankles

➤ If the casualty must be moved in order to facilitate the tending of a more serious wound or if they vomit, place them the spinal recovery position (see above)

➤ Keep the casualty warm while monitoring breathing and circulation until evacuation can be arranged.

IMPROVISED NECK COLLAR

A neck collar can be formed by placing a folded newspaper or magazine inside a large triangular bandage. Place the collar around the casualty's neck and secure. Make sure that the collar is tight enough to offer sup-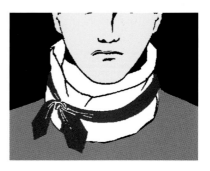port to the neck without interfering with their breathing.

Crush Injuries

In the majority of crush injuries some form of weight has fallen on the victim or the victim has been forced against an immovable object. In the first instance the fallen object may still be covering the victim and will have to be removed prior to any treatment. In the latter case it should also be fairly obvious how the crush injury occurred.

TREATMENT

The removal of any weighted object from the body of a casualty should be done with care. Be extremely careful when lifting the object, especially trees because the impact may have caused bodily impalement. Test the weight before attempting to lift the object as you may cause further damage to the casualty. Get help if available.

Once the object or casualty has been moved, perform your ABC regime (see p.22). Next examine the casualty: the crush impact area should correlate to the position of the impact object. For example, if a person has been hit by a falling tree which has landed on the chest, then check for broken ribs and signs of internal bleeding (see p.65)

Burns

A burn is damage caused to the skin by heat. Naked flames, boiling water, electrical devices, friction, acid, liquid oxygen, freezing metal and the sun all cause skin burns. The severity of the burn and the amount of body area affected will determine the casualty's survival chances. Care should be taken when dealing with severe burns to the hands, feet and facial areas, because any swelling may impede blood flow to the injured area. There is also a likelihood of infection because burns reduce the skin's protection against germs. A drop in blood pressure is also a danger, leading to shock if fluid loss is not immediately replaced.

ASSESSMENT

The more serious the burn, the greater the risk to life. This risk can be evaluated by 'degree' depending on the depth and area of the burn. A 1% burn is roughly equivalent to the surface of a hand.

Superficial

These are burns to the outer surface of the skin. They will cause some reddening, swelling and tenderness of the injured area. The affected skin is usually shed and replaced by the body's natural healing process.

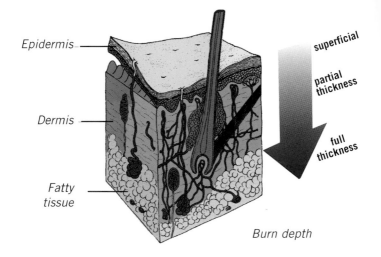

Epidermis

superficial

partial
thickness

Dermis

full
thickness

Fatty
tissue

Burn depth

Partial-thickness

These are much deeper and widespread burns that produce redness, swelling and blisters. Second-degree burns are extremely painful and susceptible to infection. These burns need careful management and a casualty must be evacuated to a medical facility where they exceed 5% of the total body area. Over time the body will renew the skin but some scarring may remain.

Full-thickness

These are burns which have penetrated through all the skin layers exposing charred muscle and bone. The skin is pale and waxy, although there may be little or no pain due to nerve damage. The skin will not recover naturally and will require skin grafts. These help promote wound recovery and prevent infection.

The Rule of Nines

The rule of nines is a division of the human body into eleven roughly equal parts of nine per cent. These parts allow us to assess the amount of body area affected by a burn (as indicated by the diagram below). Any injury covering 9% of the body surface will almost certainly require medical attention. In certain cases where the burn is deep (for example, an electrical burn), any injury to the skin larger than 2.5 cm will also require evacuation to a medical facility.

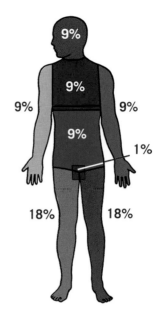

The Rule of Nines: each of the coloured areas is roughly equivalent to 9% of the body's surface area, except for each leg (18%), the entire back (18%) and the groin (1%)

TREATMENT

Perform the ABC regime (see p.22), paying particular attention to the casualty's airway and breathing in case his respiratory tract has been damaged.

Burns caused by naked flame should be cooled immediately to limit heat damage to the skin tissues. Either pour cold water slowly over the affected part, or immerse it totally in clean cold water. This should be done for at least ten minutes to stop further tissue damage and to reduce pain and swelling.

Do not attempt to remove any charred fibres that have stuck to the burn but remove any restrictive clothing around the site to prevent further swelling.

Once the burn has been cooled, a dressing should be immediately applied to limit the possibility of it becoming infected. The dressing should be sterile and made of a non-fluffy material. Avoid adhesive dressings as these will only aggravate the injury and cause more damage.

In an emergency, where several people have been burnt, clothes and sheets can be used as dressings. These can be sterilised by scorching the cloth with a candle or any naked flame in order to kill most of the bacteria. For facial injuries cut out a mask (eye, nose and mouth) and cover the head.

Burns from acids or corrosive liquids should be flushed with clean water immediately. Where the cor-rosive liquid has entered the eye, intermittent flush-ing over 20 minutes should take place. Encourage the casualty to blink or open the eye so that the water can flow over the eyeball.

Do not be tempted to burst any blisters that form, because these provide a protective layer. The only exceptions are large blisters that look like bursting, or those that contain a very milky colour which indicates possible infection. The loose skin from a ruptured burn should be cut away – this is totally painless. The area should then be covered with an antibacterial ointment and protected with a dressing.

If polythene bags are available they can be used to cover the burnt limb and help stop further infection. To reduce the possibility of shock setting in (see shock, p.68), lay the casualty down and keep them warm and comforted. If the casualty is unconscious, turn them over into the recovery position (p.30) and monitor their breathing and pulse closely. If breathing or heartbeat stop provide resuscitation immediately (see CPR, p.25).

BASIC BURNS PROCEDURES

➤ Cool the burnt area by immersion in cold clean water

➤ Flush corrosive liquids from the skin and especially the eyes

➤ Remove restricting items (clothing and watches) before the swelling starts

➤ Protect hands and feet from further infection with a sealed polythene bag

➤ Do not use adhesive or fluffy dressing

➤ Do not break blisters or remove loose skin unless necessary

➤ Do not apply ointment, oils or fats to the burn

➤ Give the casualty plenty of fluid to drink

EXTENSIVE BURNS

It should be noted that casualties with extensive burns
in excess of 75% of the body have little chance of survival. Even with a quick evacuation to an advanced
medical facility, the casualty is unlikely to survive
longer than three days.

Diseases

It is essential for travellers to find out what diseases they may be exposed to in the country or region they are visiting and how they are transmitted. Many diseases are transmitted by parasitic organisms such as mosquitoes, ticks and mites. Tropical mosquitoes transmit malaria, yellow fever, dengue fever, encephalitis and filariasis. In many cases the first sign of a disease starts with fever.

FEVER

Fever is a complex response of the body to infection and is one of the body's defence mechanisms. Fever results from a disturbance of the heat-regulating mechanism of the body by the action of toxins on the general metabolism and on the heat-regulating centre in the brain.

Humans are warm-blooded with a constant body temperature of about 37°C (98.6°F). This temperature remains almost constant despite any change in environmental surroundings. However, during a fever, body temperature can vary from anywhere between 32.2°C (90°F) to 43.3°C (110°F) and if the temperature remains at either end of this scale for any length of time, the casualty is in grave danger.

When the temperature is taken in the mouth during cold weather the thermometer should be left in for about four minutes. The temperature should never be taken immediately after a hot or cold drink. In addition to infection, a slight rise in temperature may be brought about by exercise or exposure to high temperatures.

Types of Fever

When the body becomes infected, the body's thermostatic control sets its self at a higher level in an effort to combat the invading microorganisms. The commencement of fever is usually sudden, with the person feeling hot and having flushed skin which is frequently accompanied by a rigor or shivering attack. There are three principal types of fever:

Continued fever

The temperature does not fluctuate more than 2° Fahrenheit in 24 hours and at no time reaches normal (as in typhoid).

Remittent fever

If the temperature remains above normal, but the fluctuation exceeds 2° Fahrenheit (as in TB).

Intermittent fever

If during some period of the day the temperature falls to normal or below normal, it is called intermittent fever (e.g. as in malaria).

Effects of Fever

➤   General increase in metabolic rate.

➤ Increased breakdown of the body's proteins, which can lead to weight loss if the fever is prolonged.

➤ Diminished amounts of secretions and excretions which make digestion difficult. The amount of urine is decreased.

➤ The respiration rate is increased.

➤ The circulation of blood is increased, with a rapid bounding pulse.

➤ The nervous system is affected, with high fever producing headaches and delirium.

TREATMENT

The best treatment is aspirin or paracetamol with bedrest in a well-ventilated room. If the temperature rises above 40°C (104°F) then additional cooling with fans, ice or a wet sponge may be required. Then the underlying cause must be diagnosed and treated. Give plenty of fluids to replace fluid loss and increase the amount of urine, therefore flushing the kidneys. Maintain the patient's general strength by giving plenty of easily digestible food. Continue to check pulse and temperature and treat any complications as they arise.

MALARIA

As mosquitoes breed in stagnant, sluggish water or swampy ground, you would be well advised to avoid camping near any such areas, aiming for higher ground where possible. Mosquitos bite mostly during the late evening and at night (though mosquitoes that carry dengue fever – see p. 115 – also bite during the day). The main disease spread by the mosquito is malaria. This disease is common in many parts of the world but is found mainly in the tropics and subtropics. Once infected by the mosquito bite, 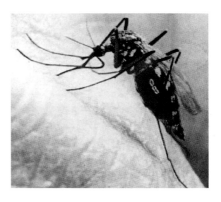 the parasites develop in the liver, progressing into the bloodstream and invading the red blood cells. The rupture of the red blood cells leads to the characteristic fever, chills and sweating associated with malaria. The cycle is sustained as the parasites from the ruptured cells invade other red blood cells. The symptoms can take weeks or even months to develop.

TREATMENT

The best protection is to start a course of anti-malarial drugs two weeks prior to any travel into an area of high risk; your doctor will be able to advise on the specific drug to use.

In the field:

➤ Use any available insect repellent.

➤ Make sure that exposed skin is covered as much as possible; tuck trouser legs into socks and sleeves into gloves. Cover your body with clothing, mosquito netting, handkerchiefs or anything else that may be improvised.

Smearing mud over any exposed areas of skin will deter the amount of mosquito bites.

If you develop an unexpected fever after your return home from the tropics you should immediately consult your doctor. Where travel is prolonged and malaria has developed, the casualty should seek treatment from a doctor as soon as possible.

DENGUE FEVER

Dengue fever is an acute disease transmitted to humans by the *Aedes* mosquito, which is found throughout the tropics. There is an incubation period of roughly five to ten days after the mosquito bite before the symptoms appear.

DENGUE FEVER SYMPTOMS

The classic form of dengue is characterized by:

➤ A sudden onset of chills and light fever.

➤ Pan behind the eyeballs whenever the head is moved.

➤ Severe pain to the back, legs and joints a few hours after the preceding symptoms.

➤ Rapid temperature increase, going as high as 40°C (104°F) and normally lasting for around three days.

The symptoms and fever stop for a short while and the body appears to return to normal. However, the fever and symptoms return announcing the second phase of the illness, normally in the form of swollen glands and a characteristic berry-like rash which often appears on the face. Classical dengue fever usually lasts no longer than a week and is never fatal, though the casualty will feel tired and depressed for some time to follow.

There is also a milder form of dengue which can last up to 72 hours and dengue hemorrhagic fever which is mainly limited to Southeast Asia. The symptoms are basically the same but for the damage to blood vessels. This is usually seen in small children or those who have suffered dengue fever several times.

TREATMENT

Patient care in the form of bedrest in a mosquito-free environment (to prevent reinfection) is a good start. Aspirin or codeine will help cope with fever, and headache or muscle pain. Fluids should be given to compensate for dehydration. Efforts should be made to protect all those around you, i.e. by using mosquito nets. Once fit to travel, the casualty should visit the nearest medical facility.

YELLOW FEVER

Yellow fever is an acute infection of the liver, kidneys and heart. It is transmitted by the female mosquito of the *Aedes* species, which breeds in pools of stagnant water.

The disease attacks in two distinct phases, with the first symptoms start developing some 3-14 days after the victim has been bitten.

YELLOW FEVER SYMPTOMS

Symptoms of the first phase:

➤ Fever

➤ Chills along with headache

➤ Backache and generalized muscle pain

➤ Nausea, vomiting

➤ Flushed face and confusion

Symptoms of the second phase:

➤ Jaundice

➤ Bleeding gums

➤ Vomiting of blood

In some cases, yellow fever produces milder effects with symptoms similar to influenza, malaria, dengue fever or typhoid. In this case, the fever generally lasts less than a week. Be aware that the first stage systems are similar to those of other diseases such as dengue fever.

TREATMENT

As with similar infections, immunization at least ten days before departure is the best prevention. Treatment for those who have contracted yellow fever involves relieving the symptoms and any additional complications. It must be stressed that most travellers who become affected suffer only mild symptoms.

However, those people who travel to an area where the disease is widespread and who have not been vaccinated put themselves at greater risk. Yellow fever occurs predominately in South America, the Caribbean Islands and Africa. The frequency of the disease increases in the summer as the mosquito population swells, but it occurs year round in tropical climates.

RESPIRATORY DISEASES

The 'common cold' affects the upper respiratory system and is the most widespread of all infectious diseases. This viral infection is transmitted by the inhalation of microscopic droplets, usually from a person sneezing next to you. A 'cold' is in fact a term used to describe any illness caused by one or a combination of over a hundred viruses which all produce similar symptoms. The duration and intensity of the common cold vary considerably, but on average the illness will resolve itself within a week. The precise symptoms vary from one person to the next but sneezing, headache and varying degree of malaise are usually experienced.

TREATMENT

You cannot cure a cold but its symptoms can be relieved. Bed rest and inducing sweating by the use of blankets, for example, as well as hot drinks and drugs, such as aspirin, can be used to relieve headaches. The use of decongestants, antihistamines and cough suppressants can also be beneficial. Persistent and developing symptoms may indicate a more serious illness is developing.

TUBERCULOSIS

Tuberculosis (or TB) is disease of the lungs - although any organ in the body may be infected – caused by the tubercle bacillus. Two varieties of the tubercle bacillus are found in humans: the human variety which is largely responsible for pulmonary TB, and the bovine (derived from cows) which causes most cases of bone and glandular TB. Both produce their effect on the body by the formation of the same type of specialized granulation tissue. The human type is more common in towns while the bovine type is more common in rural areas. Tuberculosis is mainly contracted by exposure to infected individuals, especially during their habitual bouts of coughing.

In addition to the local lung damage, toxins produced by the bacilli are absorbed into the general circulation, producing a profound effect on the metabolic processes of the body, including fever, rapid pulse, sweating and loss of weight. When the individual manufactures sufficient antibodies to limit the local activity of the disease and to neutralize the circulating toxins, there is improvement in these general symptoms.

TREATMENT

There is no immediate threat to the traveller, although there are an increasing number of cases of TB that are proving to be resistant to the current anti-tuberculosis medications. Most of these resistant cases have been found in patients who have AIDS. The symptoms are non-specific and normally mild, including cough, malaise, weight-loss and low-grade fever. TB is not a life-threatening illness in the early stages, although any traveller who has spent time in a area where the disease is prevalent should take precautions and consult their doctor upon returning home.

PNEUMONIA

There are a number of different types of pneumonia but for the purposes of this book, the simplest distinction is between bacterial pneumonia and viral pneumonia. Bacterial pneumonia is usually an acute primary infection occurring in a previously healthy respiratory tract, while viral pneumonia is often secondary to other conditions such as bronchitis, aspiration of foreign or infected material, blockage of a bronchus or congestion of the lungs.

BACTERIAL PNEUMONIA SYMPTOMS

➤ Chills with the abrupt onset of fever, sometimes accompanied by a rigor or vomiting.

➤ The tongue is furred

➤ The pulse and respiration rates are raised

➤ A short dry cough, later accompanied by the characteristic 'rusty' phlegm

➤ Pain in the chest, which is worse on coughing and deep breathing, is common.

(Cont'd)

- ➤ Development of groups of small blisters about the mouth and lips
- ➤ Flushing of the cheeks, which is often more marked on the same side as the affected lung, together with blue tinges to the lips and ears may be present

The symptoms of viral pneumonia are very similar, but they are less severe and the onset is more gradual.

TREATMENT

There is little to be done to treat pneumonia in the field. However, the condition does not pose an immediate threat to life and if the evacuation is prolonged, you should place the casualty in plenty of fresh air. Continue to check the airway. Disturb them as little as possible and let them rest in a position that is comfortable. Encourage them to eat and drink as much as possible.

TYPHUS

Typhus is an infectious disease transmitted to humans by lice. The incubation period between infection and the onset of symptoms is two weeks. The disease is abrupt, with fever (40°C, 104°F) and severe headache resulting in delirium and confusion. A pinkish rash appears a few days later which over the course of the disease turns to dark red. Blood pressure is normally low and there may be signs of pneumonia (see opposite) If untreated, the casualty will slide into unconsciousness and possibly die. The survival rate of those infected with typhus depends on the health and age of the casualty.

TREATMENT

Vaccination is available for those travelling through areas where the disease exists. However, good personal hygiene and the liberal use of delousing power will help prevent contamination.

BUBONIC PLAGUE

Plague is an infection transmitted to humans by rodent flea bites. It is particularly rampant in Asia, especially Cambodia and the surrounding countries. The incubation period is two to ten days with the first symptoms being the sudden onset of a high fever, severe headache, general muscle ache and malaise. In areas where an epidemic has occurred, the casualty may become severely septic with open sores and spots appearing on the skin. By this stage the casualty is usually comatose.

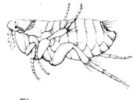

Flea

TREATMENT

You should isolate those with suspected plague, especially those that are coughing as this spreads the disease. Those in attendance should take every care not to become infected. Where plague is confirmed, seek advice before requesting an evacuation.

MENINGITIS

Meningitis can be a life-threatening disease which causes inflammation of the membranes surrounding the brain. Either viruses or bacteria may cause the inflammation. The microorganisms which cause meningitis enter from either an external source (head wound) or and internal source such as an upper respiratory infection. The disease is found world-wide especially in Africa and India. Those persons infected can spread the disease through coughs and sneezing.

All forms of meningitis regardless of their cause share a number of common symptoms.

MENINGITIS SYMPTOMS

➤ A headache which increases in intensity
➤ A high fever and stiffness of the neck
➤ A sore throat
➤ Nausea and vomiting

The progressive disease brings drowsiness, delirium and possibly coma. At this stage the eyes can become very sensitive to light.

TREATMENT

Little can be done to treat the disease in the field as

definitive diagnosis will depend on studying the cerebrospinal fluid. Any suspect casualty should be evacuated to a medical facility as soon as possible.

INFECTIOUS HEPATITIS

This is a viral infection of the liver. There are five different types of viral hepatitis but in this book we will deal with the two basic forms, hepatitis A and hepatitis B. Although the symptoms of both are very similar there is a difference in length of incubation and the means by which the virus is spread. Hepatitis B is mainly transmitted through blood-to-blood contact, for example during sex or by the sharing of syringes by drug users. The virus for hepatitis A is found in faeces and is usually transmitted by contaminated food and water, though it can also be blood-borne. The incubation period for hepatitis A is about four weeks, while the symptoms for hepatitis B can take anywhere from 6 to 12 weeks to develop. In many people hepatitis will go unnoticed.

In both cases the common symptoms will be headache, fever, nausea and vomiting accompanied by aching of the muscles. Within five to ten days the patient develops jaundice, causing a yellowing of the skin (though it should be noted that some patients never develop jaundice). At this stage the symptoms increase slightly before falling back after 24 hours. The liver may become enlarged and tender.

TREATMENT

In the wilderness it is only possible to cope with uncomplicated cases, which means bed rest and the safe removal of the patient's infected excreta and sterilisation of utensils. Fluids should be given if vomiting is excessive. The casualty should avoid exercise and not be given any alcohol. Strict isolation is not necessary. Due to the long incubation period, it is more likely that most travellers will have returned home before the symptoms develop.

Food & Water Contamination Diseases

A major health threat to any traveller is the danger of infection through consuming contaminated food or water. Most Western countries have strict food hygiene standards and stomach upsets are rarely serious. Unfortunately, the same cannot be said for the poorer nations where food and water can be extremely scarce. Even where food is plentiful, washing plates and cooking utensils in a monsoon dish hardly constitutes proper hygiene.

The human body is made up of around 70 per cent water and we cannot survive without water longer than four days in a hot climate and 12 in a cold one. In a temperate climate, while carrying out a normal level of activity, the body requires a daily fluid intake of 2.5 litres (4.5 pints). This requirement fluctuates according to the humidity, air temperature and physical activity. Not only is the quantity of water important, it's quality is also vital. Contaminated or impure water will cause the traveller more harm than good, increasing water loss and the risk of serious disease. Although waterborne diseases pose a great health risk to the traveller, this needs to be balanced against the body's natural demand for fluids.

FRESH DRINKABLE WATER SOURCES

Rain, streams and rivers provide the majority of the world's drinkable water. Unfortunately, where there is human habitation, much of it becomes contaminated before we get to drink it. Water infected with faeces and urine can cause, amongst other things, dysentery, cholera and typhoid. Fresh water is often available in bottled form but this can be expensive in some coun- 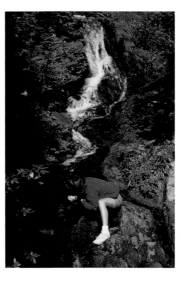 tries. An easier way to obtain clean water therefore is to filter and sterilise it.

Filtering and Sterilisation

Filtering will remove mud particles, plant matter and small waterborne creatures, and sterilisation will kill off almost all infectious germs. There are many filtering systems on the market, most of which are aimed at the individual traveller. Some both filter and sterilise. (see overleaf)

Sterilisation can be achieved by boiling water vigorously for at least ten minutes. Make sure that the heat is

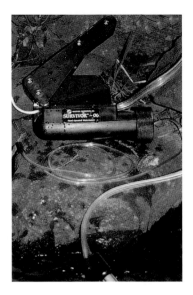

Portable water filter

distributed evenly by having it on a rolling boil. Provided the water has been well boiled the colour and taste are of no consequence. Another method is chemical sterilisation, such as chlorine-based purification tablets, potassium permanganate and iodine. Be sure to follow the instructions carefully. Chemical sterilisation tends to leave an unpleasant taste and odour in the water, and both the iodine and potassium will stain the water pink.

SAS ACTION

➤ In the SAS the problem of drinking contaminated water is partially overcome by drinking tea or coffee which automatically requires boiling water in the preparation. The less contamination you let past your mouth the less chance of infection.

DANGEROUS WATERING HOLES

When eating or drinking in foreign cities and towns always give the toilets a quick inspection. While they may not be modern they should at least be clean. A dirty toilet indicates a dirty establishment. Where you are forced to squat over an open hole, it is more likely that you will grip the walls with your hands, so wash them thoroughly afterwards. Also, locally prepared drinks, milk, ice and ice cream should all be treated as suspect, as they are only as pure as the water they are made from. This is particularly so in the tropical countries.

In the wilderness, animal bones in the vicinity of stagnant pools could mean the water is poisonous, so always sterilise or if possible distil before drinking. Approach any isolated watering hole with caution

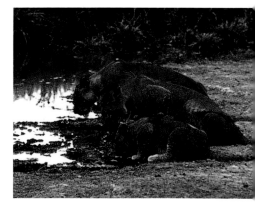

as this will be visited by a variety of animals, including predators.

CONTAMINATION DISEASES

Diarrhoea

Most people who travel to a foreign land will suffer from bouts of diarrhoea. Although unpleasant they

SAS ACTION

➤ Once while serving with the SAS in Northern Malaya I went to the local village of Grik for a meal. I had several bottles of beer and a Nasi Goring (a mixture of rice, vegetables and fish), the latter I watched being cooked in a very hot wok. The problem was I finished up having a locally made ice cream. I returned to camp and went to bed. At around two in the morning I was woken with the most terrible stomach pain and a desperate need to use the toilet (I actually leapt from the camp bed and dived through an open window, this being the shortest course to the latrines). I suffered terribly for the next 24 hours until the patrol medic gave me the antibiotic tetracycline, which stopped the bacteria in its tracks.

pose no threat to life and the disorder is usually self-limiting. In the case of the average traveller, diarrhoea is usually caused by the change in diet, or less likely as a result of consuming contaminated food or water, although malaria, cholera and salmonella produce a similar disorder. Diarrhoea is detected when the number of daily bowel movements are increased by a factor of two or more, with stools being squishy and watery. Nausea and vomiting are frequently caused by infections of the stomach or intestines, which are often viral so antibiotics are of no value. These infections will usually resolve without treatment in 24 to 48 hours.

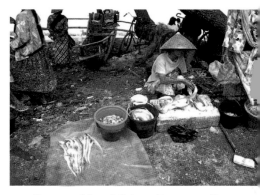

Beware of local fish as they are often the cause of stomach upsets

TREATMENT

Water loss must be replaced using sterile water (boiled) mixed with a little salt. Check medical packs for any electrolyte powders. If you have none of these, a small amount of pulverized charcoal taken from a cold fire and swallowed with some water will settle the stomach. A juice made from potassium-rich fruit, such as apples and oranges, will also help, as will honey if it can be found.

Dysentery

Dysentery is an infection of the large gut caused by bacteria or amoebic infection. This is most often the result of poor personal hygiene in the preparation or handling of food. Flies also spread the infection, and some infected people can act as carriers while showing no signs of having the disease. The diarrhoea is painful with the stools containing blood and mucus.

Symptoms can appear anywhere from 30 minutes to 12 hours after consuming contaminated food and range from mild stomach upset with loose stools to the rapid onset of rigorous and painful cramps with acute bloody diarrhoea. The casualty may also feel nauseous but rarely vomits. A rarer form of the disease, amoebic dysentery, sometimes takes three or four weeks to develop. Bowl movements involve much straining and the stools are foul-smelling and increasingly stained with blood.

TREATMENT

As with any infection, treatment will depend on the severity, but most dysentery symptoms will disappear within 24 to 36 hours. Mild cases can be treated with kaolin while the more serious casualties of dysentery will need antibiotic treatment. In all cases the need for replacing body fluid and salt is essential.

Cholera

Cholera is an infectious disease and is most widespread in the Middle East, Asia and Africa. The illness is transmitted through water, seafoods and other foods

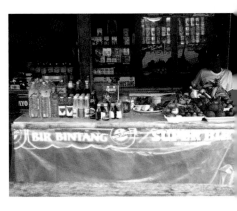

Peeling fresh fruit and drinking bottled water will help prevent many diseases

that have been contaminated by the excrement of an infected person.

Those infected with cholera will start to feel the effects (which can be explosive) anywhere from a few hours to several days. The first symptom is normally diarrhoea, the stools of which are grey and watery with little sign of normal faecal matter. These are almost continuous, resulting in a dangerously high fluid loss. There may also be some vomiting, and urine output will almost cease. In mild cases complete recovery can occur within a week, while the more severe cases can cause death within 48 hours.

TREATMENT

Although immunization is available, it is only partially protective, and in addition it requires two injections up to six weeks apart with a booster every three months. The best line of defence is to be wary of what you eat and drink. Make sure everything is fresh and clean – then check your own hands.

The management of cholera requires bed rest and the replacement of fluids and salts lost through diarrhoea. If the disease is recognized early, then the water can be given by mouth; however, in severe cases fluid has to be given by direct infusion into a vein. Antibiotics such as tetracycline will help fight the bacteria.

Typhoid

A bacterial infection acquired from consuming food and water contaminated by human sewage containing the organism Salmonella typhosa. It is also found in dairy produce and uncooked meats. Typhoid was once one of the most dangerous fevers affecting humans and to this day it remains a threat in countries with low standards of hygiene and inadequate sanitation. The source of most infections are chronic carriers with a continual urinary tract contagion. Tourists and travellers still die from the disease once they have returned home. The incubation period is anywhere between one to two weeks, though symptoms may not start for some five weeks after eating contaminated food.

At the onset there may be headaches, fever, a general loss of energy and malaise. A cough is common which may be accompanied by a sore throat and nose bleed. There is frequently abdominal pain, constipation and vomiting. Within a week the casualty grows weaker as the fever steadily increases on a daily basis, causing confusion and delirium. By this stage the casualty becomes very sick with severe diarrhoea or constipation while the abdomen starts to swell. During the second or third week a pink rash appears, heralding the onset of serious complications including the perforation or haemorrhaging of the intestine. The temperature rises on a daily basis for the first week, often as high as 40°C (104°F), though the pulse may remain only slightly above normal. Luckily, the fever starts to subside at this stage leading to a normal recovery for most people.

TREATMENT

Vaccination provides the best protection. For those

who have already contracted typhoid, an early diagnosis will help and a course of antibiotics is usually administered. In all cases, the replacement of fluid loss is essential, especially if there has been diarrhoea (usually in the latter stages of the disease). In the wilderness, pay strict attention to the removal of contaminated stools and urine.

Botulism

This is a serious life-threatening illness caused by the bacteria *Clostridium botulinum*. This bacteria is found in soil and watery environments, such as sea water, and also in fish and other animals. Humans normally acquire the disease from contaminated food which has not been cooked or heated properly. The organism is only killed after the food has been heated to 121°C (250°F).

Once inside the body the toxin produced by the bactria is quickly absorbed producing gastrointestinal symptoms of abdominal pain, nausea and vomiting. This is followed by an attack on the nervous system which results in blurred vision, difficulty in swallowing and muscular weakness, especially in the arms and legs. Finally the toxin attacks the respiratory system, paralysing the muscles used for breathing. Bilateral dilated, unreactive pupils is a common sign in many botulism cases. The incubation period from time of ingestion to the onset of the symptoms is 18–36 hours.

Botulism can also be absorbed through open wounds (including minor cuts). The symptoms take longer to develop, normally around ten days, and are similar to those of food botulism but without gastrointestinal indications.

TREATMENT

The illness produces a wide variety of conditions from a mild stomach upset to death. In the most serious cases, preservation of the respiratory system must have priority. Those persons suspected of being contaminated with the botulism toxin must have immediate evacuation to a medical facility, preferably one with a respirator. If the source originated from contaminated food then purgative treatment and enemas may also prove useful.

Schistosomiasis (bilharziasis)

More than 200 million people worldwide are infected with schistosomiasis, more commonly called bilharziasis. It causes ill health, lethargy and death. This is an illness caused by parasitic worms which actively seek and penetrate the skin of any humans bathing in infected fresh water. Once in the human bloodstream they move firstly to the lungs before migrating to the area of the liver and bladder. As the worms proliferate, the patient may have repeated attacks of diarrhoea and blood may also be seen in the urine. If left untreated, this can lead to either liver or kidney failure.

Symptoms are fever with malaise. The casualty may also have a red itchy rash, diarrhoea, and abdominal or urinary tract pain. Loss of appetite and weight are also common, and there is often bladder pain and blood in the urine. In many cases bilharziasis may cause few or no symptoms and requires no immediate medical attention. However, if you have visited an area where bilharziasis is endemic you are advised to have a medical check-up upon your return. The risk can be reduced if you avoid swimming in water which is infested with snails. Large rivers and lakes such as the Nile, Euphrates and Lake Victoria are badly infected.

TREATMENT

Bilharziasis is often confused with dysentery (see p.131), so if the casualty does not respond to treatment for normal gastrointestinal disorders, then bilharziasis should be suspected. A conclusive diagnosis is dependent on finding the worm eggs in the stools. There is no vaccine available to combat bilharziasis, but drugs such as praziquantel are very effective in dealing with the worms. Those with suspected bilharziasis should have a check-up upon their return home.

POISONING

There are various forms of poison, and depending on the quantity taken into the body, many can result in death. Poisons can enter the body through the mouth either by eating or drinking, through the inhalation of gases or by absorption through the skin. The primary forms of poisoning include carbon monoxide gas (see p.41), ingestion of household or industrial products, drugs, alcohol, bites and food.

It is essential to determine the type of poisoning.

Where a casualty has been bitten by an insect or snake the cause is fairly self-evident. In all other cases you should establish what has been ingested, whether chemicals, alcohol, fungi etc. How much time has elapsed since ingestion? How much of the substance was ingested and what reaction has it had on the casualty?

POISONING POINTERS

➤ Skin colouration – a flushed red skin may indicate carbon monoxide poisoning

➤ Smell the casualty's breath for alcohol or petroleum-based products

➤ Check for burning or reddening around the mouth

➤ Has the casualty vomited?

➤ Is there an empty container nearby?

➤ Has the casualty had a drink or just eaten a meal?

TREATMENT

The first priority to perform the ABC regime (see p.22), particularly with regard maintaining a clear airway: a sleepy or unconscious casualty risks asphyxia. If the casualty is vomiting voluntarily, they should be left to continue, but as a rule of thumb – apart from poisonous plant ingestion or drug overdose – vomiting should **not** be induced.

Alkalis (such as bleach and ammonia) Give diluted citrus

fruit juice or vinegar mixed 50/50 with water.

Kerosene, gasoline etc. If small amounts have been taken, do not induce vomiting. Protect the airway. Give 100 per cent oxygen if available and monitor the heart rhythm. When more than 50 ml ($1^3/_4$ fl oz) of a petroleum product have been swallowed then vomiting should be induced as this amount poses a serious threat to the brain and heart.

Strong domestic acids Give milk, egg white or flour mixed in water and these may help neutralize and dilute the acid.

Methanol-based alcohol products Give a small shot of ethanol-based alcohol every hour as this inhibits the metabolization of methanol.

In all cases it is essential to keep the airway open and monitor the heart rhythm. Those casualties who are unconscious should be placed in the recovery position (see p.29). Where large quantities or strong poisons have been taken the casualty should be evacuated immediately to a medical facility.

Plant Poisoning

For those travelling in the wilderness, the main form of poisoning comes from poorly prepared or contaminated food. However, many travellers also put themselves at risk when they experiment by eating wild plants, which only increases the chances of being poisoned. This danger can be averted by eating only those plants or fungi that are easily recognisable or, for plants only, by carrying out an edibility test. It is well worth learning in advance of a trip how to identify edible and inedible plants in the the areas in which you will be travelling.

Plants Poisons

There are two fairly common plant poisons which are worth learning how to identify:

➤ *Hydrocyanic acid* This tastes and smells of peaches or bitter almonds and can be tested for by crushing leaves.

➤ *Oxalic acid* This can be identified from the burning or stinging sensation when crushed parts of the plant are rubbed on the skin.

All plants with either characteristic should **not** be eaten under any circumstance.

A selection of poisonous plant, fungi and fruits are illustrated on pages 141 and 142.

POISONOUS PLANTS

Plants showing any of the following characteristics should be avoided unless positively identified as a species that is safe to eat:

➤ a milky sap

➤ red colouring

➤ fruit divided into five segments

➤ grasses with small barbs on the leaves

➤ wilted or old leaves

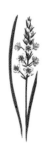

Death Camas
(N. America)

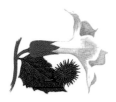

Thorn apple or
Jimson weed
(Temperate regions
and Tropics)

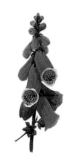

Foxglove

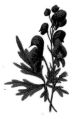

Monk's Hood

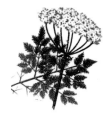

Hemlock

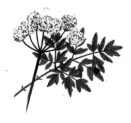

Water hemlock
or Cowbanes

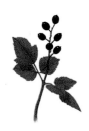

Bane berries

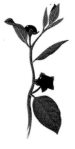

Deadly
Nightshade

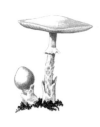

Destroying Angel
(Amanita virosa)

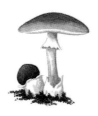

Death cap
(Amanita phalloides)

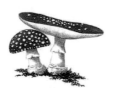

Panther Cap
(Amanita pantheri-
na)

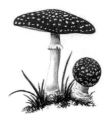

Fly agaric
(Amanita muscaria)

Leaden entoloma
(Entoloma sinnuatum)

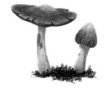

Inocybe patouillardii

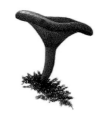

Paxilus involatus

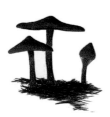

Cortinarius
speciosissimus

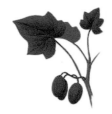

Physic nut
(Tropics)

Strychnine
(Tropics)

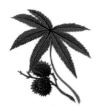

Castor Oil
plant
(Tropics)

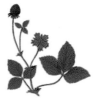

Duchesnia
(Tropics)

Edibility Test

A plant's identity must be 100% established. If for any reason you are at all unsure whether it is edible or not, follow these simple steps below. Be thorough in your testing and test only one plant with one person at a time so that any effects can be properly monitored.

WARNING

➤ The plant edibility test will not work for fungi.

GENERAL RULES

➤ Avoid collecting plants from any area which may have been contaminated and those with milky saps (except for dandelion, goat's beard and coconut) or any of the other characteristics listed above. Wash any plant material thoroughly before cooking and remove any diseased or damaged parts.

➤ Not all the parts of any one plant may be edible. Separate the root, stem, leaves and any fruit and test each part separately.

➤ Only test plants that are plentiful in the environment you are in. There is no point in subjecting your body to possible poisoning if there is only a handful of the plant available.

CONDUCTING THE TEST

➤ First test the plant for any contact poisons. Crush

a leaf and rub a little of the sap onto the sensitive skin of the inner wrist. If after 15 minutes no itching, blistering or burning has occurred, continue.

➤ Take a small portion of crushed plant and place it in your mouth between your gum and lower lip. Leave it for five minutes. If there are no 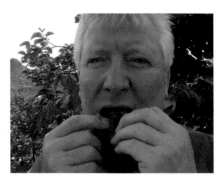 unpleasant reactions, chew the plant and note whether it exhibits any disagreeable properties such as burning, extreme bitterness or a soapy taste. If it still seems all right, swallow down the juice but spit out the pulp. Allow eight hours to pass to see if any adverse effects develop, such as sickness, dizziness, sleepiness, stomach aches or cramps.

➤ If none occur, take a slightly larger amount, such as a teaspoonful, and wait for another eight hours.

➤ If there are still no problems, eat a handful of the plant and wait for a further 24 hours. If after this time, the plant has given you no ill effects, you can assume that it is safe and can be eaten in greater quantities.

TREATMENT

If plant poisoning is suspected, the casualty must be

encouraged to vomit. A glass of water mixed with salt followed rapidly by gagging should produce the desired result. Use your fingers or a smooth cold instrument such as a spoon handle to stimulate the throat. After vomiting is completed, give the casualty a drink of charcoal slurry which should help absorb any remaining poison.

Check breathing and pulse and resuscitate if necessary. If the casualty is unconscious place them in the recovery position (p. 00).

AUTHOR'S NOTE

➤ Many medical books advise not to induce vomiting. This is certainly the correct advice where toxic or corrosive substances have been ingested, but not with poisonous plants. The release of poison from a plant, or fruit is much slower, therefore vomiting will greatly reduce the amount of poison absorbed into the blood system.

Environmental Medical Problems

It must be stressed that environmental medical problems do not stem from the weather (i.e. temperature differences) alone; along with the cold and heat, come dangerous obstacles and the rigours of the wilderness, including rivers, lightning, flash floods and so on.

Providing you are equipped with the appropriate clothing, the body will adjust to most environments. On average, it takes about two weeks for the body to acclimatise fully to the heat of the desert, or the cold of the Arctic. However, even when acclimatised, environmental risks are still present. A traveller in the desert will need an adequate supply of water, while in the cold the need is to stay warm. Walking in either the heat or cold can exhaust both physical and mental reserves, so a strong, positive attitude is needed.

The human body functions best at temperatures around 37°C (98.6°F). It maintains this temperature in all environments by conduction/convection, radiation and sweating. Sweating, the most important of these processes, cools the body when the water on the skin evaporates. Of course, if you are in an area where the humidity is high, the sweat will not evaporate easily and you will have the worst of all scenarios: loss of bodily fluids and an increase in body heat. Sweating in a cold environment is not a good idea, because when you cease to exercise the sweat may freeze.

HOT AREAS

The intense heat of a desert is a threat to the body's ability to regulate its temperature. The human body is made up of 75 per cent water, and it is essential for this amount of fluid to be maintained by the body for it to work properly. A loss of two pints will seriously decrease efficiency by 25 per cent. Once the body's cooling system has been compromised, heat exhaustion, or heat-stroke, will occur and may be fatal. Also, lack of salt will cause heat cramps. Therefore, ensuring adequate water, food and salt intake will lessen the risk of suffering these debilitating and potentially deadly conditions.

In the day, temperatures in the desert can soar to 58°C (136° F), but by contrast the night-time temperatures, especially in the northern Gobi and Siberian deserts, can 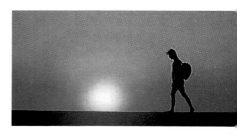 fall as low as minus 50 degrees Fahrenheit. These may also be accompanied by strong winds which will increase the wind-chill factor. It may seem strange that a place that can be so hot in the day becomes so cold at night. In the day the sun gives out heat which is absorbed by the sand, gravel or rocks of the desert. At night, this heat radiates back into the sky. Without any clouds to contain it, it escapes into the upper atmosphere, therefore causing the desert to lose heat and cool rapidly.

Dehydration

Arid regions are those least likely to have an easily available source of water. The traveller must make sure that adequate supplies of fresh water are available. Dehydration is a slow process that occurs when the loss of bodily fluid is greater than that replacing it. Any permanent or semi-permanent water source in a desert, such as an oasis or a well, is a rare and treasured resource for the local

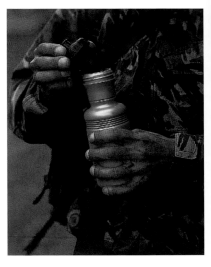

Always ensure that you carry adequate supplies of fresh water with you

population. Some deserts, where there is a high level of precipitation, have a permanent river flowing through them. Rivers such as the Nile and the Colorado are able to keep flowing because the amount of water feeding them off the surrounding desert is greater than the rate of evaporation.

Radiant Light

This is, of course, produced by the sun, but does not necessarily come from just the sun's direction. Sunlight can also be reflected off the ground and

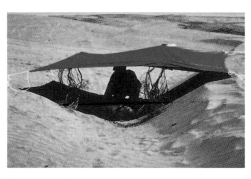

In areas of bright sunshine, protect yourself from radiant light

any nearby rocks. The light from the sun contains particles of radiation that are harmful to both skin and eyes, so both need to be protected as much as possible by light clothing and sunglasses or a hat.

Sunburn

Sunburn is the most common type of injury encountered while travelling across a desert environment. This is caused by direct and excessive exposure to the sun's rays. The effects can become even more pronounced when combined with either water (sea water or sweat in particular) or a persistent wind.

TREATMENT

Use a sun block on all exposed skin when travelling over open areas such as the desert. A wide-brimmed hat with a neck flap is also a good idea. The immediate priority in cases of sunburn is to get the casualty out of the sun immediately and protect him from further exposure. Cool the burnt area with calamine or similar soothing lotion. If these are not available, sponge with cold water. Treat any burn blisters (see Burns, p.107) to prevent the possibility of infection. The casualty will be severely dehydrated, so make sure that they drink plenty of fluids and gets plenty of rest.

Desert Cold

The desert is a place of immense temperature contrast, and while the heat can be overwhelming during the day, the nights can become intensely cold. Lack of the right clothing or shelter will, again, threaten the body's ability to control its temperature and may well result in hypothermia or frostbite. Remember that any wind will increase the chill factor and make any temperature loss even greater. During the evening, as the air chills, more layers of clothing should be added as necessary. As the air heats up again in the morning,

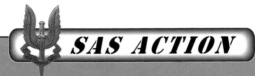

SAS ACTION

➤ During the Gulf war several members of the SAS operating behind the Iraqi lines were spotted by the enemy and forced to carry out escape and evasion tactics. This involved travelling vast distance at night through the worst weather the region had seen for many years. All suffered from varying degrees of hypothermia, and one even died from it.

they should be gradually removed. On no account should the traveller ignore the danger of hypothermia (see p.156) due to the cold desert nights.

COLD AREAS

There has been a large increase in arctic travel over the past few years as people fulfil their desire to explore these vast wildernesses. Arctic temperatures present their own problems, mainly frostbite and hypothermia.

Body Cooling

The influence of cold temperatures varies from person to person depending on age, health and protective clothing. Early signs of cold collapse start with a slowing of the individual; this is followed by stumbling and frequent falls. Symptoms range from apathy, to faked confidence or even aggression. If untreated, a fall in the body's core temperature and a

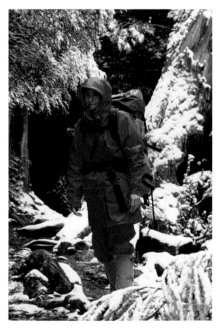

The correct clothing is the essential first step in protecting yourself against the effects of body cooling

reduction in the blood sugar level will cause total collapse and a loss of consciousness. If the core temperature is allowed to fall below 35°C (95°F) the brain will cease to function, ultimately resulting in death.

Wind will accelerate the cooling of the body because its movement markedly decreases air temperature. Being wet also increases body cooling as water con-

SAS ACTION

➤ During a winter exercise in Norway myself and five other SAS men were caught in a snow storm with high winds and low temperatures. This forced us to dig snow holes and sit out the storm. After two days the decision was made to move to lower ground. However, in order to do this we had to first climb and cross a saddle in the mountains. One of the men (who was exceptionally fit) had not been wearing the correct clothing and became extremely cold. In addition to this another man fell and broke his leg. The accumulation of fighting the freezing conditions and attending to the two casualties placed a tremendous strain on the rest of the party. Having built a sledge from a set of skis, we eventually managed to pull the two men to safety.

ducts heat away from the body, therefore cooling it rapidly. Garments that are wet or damp, either through water or sweat will lose their insulating properties and will begin to drain heat from the body.

Preparation is the key to preventing body cooling, with good waterproof clothing and extra protection for the head, hands and feet being essential.

Hands and Feet

Hands and feet are at the extremes of the body's circulation and so need extra attention if they are to maintain their heat. Make sure that any fastenings at the wrists, ankles, neck and waist are snug enough to prevent heat loss but not so tight that they cut off circulation. As much as possible, keep the hands covered. If they become cold, warm them either between the thighs or under the armpits.

Moving the feet and wiggling the toes can warm frost-nipped toes, and warming them against a companion's body is also very effective (right). Pay attention to your footwear and try to keep your feet as dry

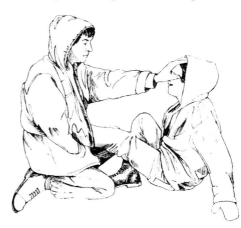

Use body heat to warm the hands and feet of those suffering from exposure

as possible. If you have a pair of spare socks, keep them close to your body and try to change into a dry pair at least once a day. Over boots are also a great aid in protecting the feet against the cold and wet. If

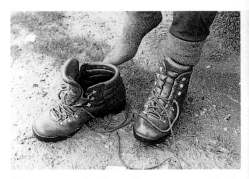

Remove your boots and massage your feet and toes while resting to ensure good circulation and so prevent frost nip

you do not have any, try and improvise by putting a spare sock over each boot. If you are not moving around, take off your boots and give your feet a good ten-minute massage every few hours.

Frostbite

When the body becomes cold, it puts priority on retaining the core heat rather than warming the extremities. Therefore it shuts down the blood vessels in the skin. In extreme cold weather, the parts of the body at the limits of the circulation (typically, the feet, hands and face) may actually freeze and cause tissue damage. This is the condition known as frostbite and can vary in severity from affecting only the skin surface to penetrating underlying tissue and fat. Frostbite can creep up on a person so gradually that they are not aware that they have it until it is well established. You will need to be on guard against this dangerous condition because if it becomes serious it can lead to gangrene and loss of the affected part.

FROSTBITE SYMPTOMS

➤ A feeling of 'pins and needles' in the affected part
➤ A subsequent stiffness and numbness
➤ The skin of the affected area will turn pale, then white, before becoming a mottled blue and eventually black as tissue death occurs

As exposed skin is most prone to frostbite, check uncovered areas frequently, especially the nose, fingers and toes. Other areas that need to be checked are the ankles and wrists. If you are with someone else, make sure that you check each other frequently for any warning signs that frostbite is occurring.

TREATMENT

If any frostbitten areas are discovered:

➤ Warm the affected part by some natural means; skin-to-skin contact provides the best method of slow warming. Use warm water if available, but make sure that it isn't too warm (above 40°C, 104°F).

➤ Remove the casualty to a shelter as soon as is practicable and insulate against further heat loss with blankets and extra clothing.

➤ Elevate any of the limbs to above heart level to minimise swelling

➤ Hot drinks and food should be given as soon as possible.

FROSTBITE

➤ DO NOT allow a thawed part to refreeze

➤ DO NOT rub or massage the affected area (except in the very early stages)

➤ DO NOT use direct or strong heat such as hot stones or a fire to warm an area

➤ DO NOT give alcohol to drink as this can lower body temperature further

➤ DO NOT allow a casualty with a recently frostbitten foot to walk

➤ DO NOT break open any blisters which may occur

Hypothermia

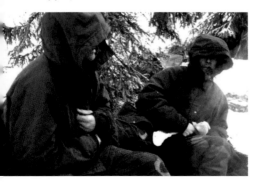

Hypothermia occurs when the body temperature falls below 35°C (95°F) and body heat is being lost faster than it can be replaced. At this stage body functions start to slow down and may stop altogether if the condition is not treated. Exposure to cold, wet weather is a major factor in this condition as is wet clothing, immersion in cold water, inadequate clothing, exhaustion and shortage of food and drink. It is important to be aware of the symptoms, especially if you are subject to any of the conditions described above.

HYPOTHERMIA SYMPTOMS

➤ Uncontrollable shivering
➤ Skin is pale and dry and abnormally cold to the touch
➤ Muscular weakness, tiredness and lethargy.
➤ Irrational behaviour
➤ A change in personality – extrovert may become introvert, a quiet person may become aggressive
➤ Dimming of sight and needing to sleep
➤ Slow, weak pulse
➤ Slow, shallow breathing
➤ Eventual collapse and unconsciousness and possible cardiac arrest

TREATMENT

As soon as hypothermia is suspected, it must be treated by restoring lost body heat (see Warming a Body, p.158). This means getting the casualty out of the wet and cold and into shelter as soon as possible. Use dry clothing or coverings to replace any wet clothing.

If the victim has been totally submerged in water, remove all the clothes because they will reduce body temperature faster than naked flesh.

If the casualty becomes unconscious with no signs of breathing or pulse, proceed immediately with the ABC regime, giving assisted ventilation and chest compression as necessary (see p.22). The casualty will still need to be warmed. Even if the casualty's body temperature has fallen to 26°C (79°F), do not automatically presume that they are dead. Carry on with resuscitation techniques until they have reached normal body temperature; if they cannot then be revived, death can be assumed.

Remember, if one person is suffering from hypothermia there maybe others so check everyone in your party.

Warming a Body

The treatment of hypothermia is centred on stopping the loss of body heat and replacing lost warmth. This is best done by sharing the body heat of a fit person (more than one if numbers allow) in a sheltered environment.

➤ Provide shelter from the wind and cold as soon as possible.

➤ If dry clothing or covering is available, use it to replace any wet clothing. Replace wet clothing in stages, uncovering as little of the body as possible at any one time. Allow even that part to remain uncovered for as brief a period as practicable.

➤ If no dry clothing is available, leave any wet garments on and cover them with additional insulation against the cold. Add a final waterproof layer. A metallised emergency blanket is ideal for this purpose. It is wind and waterproof as well as being reflective of radiated body heat.

➤ Provide body warmth. Direct person-to-person heat from another healthy traveller is particularly effective, especially in a survival or sleeping bag. However, other heat sources can be used, such as heating pads, containers of warm water, and heated rocks; none of these should be placed directly in contact with the casualty's skin.

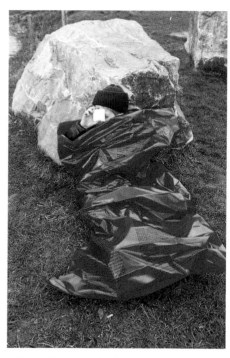

Place the casualty in a survival bag and provide external heat to warm them

➤ If the casualty is conscious, give hot, sweet food and drink.

➤ Handle the casualty gently. Frozen skin and flesh are very easily damaged.

HYPOTHERMIA

➤ DO NOT rub or massage to stimulate circulation
➤ DO NOT warm the casualty too quickly
➤ DO NOT permit the casualty further exertion
➤ DO NOT give the casualty alcohol
➤ DO NOT leave the casualty alone

Immersion Foot

If you are travelling across the wet ground such as the Arctic tundra during spring/summer your feet can be immersed in cold water or bog for a long time. If the feet are not adequately protected, they will develop a condition commonly referred to as 'immersion foot'.

IMMERSION FOOT SYMPTOMS

➤ The foot becomes white and numb, cold and swollen
➤ Subsequently, the skin becomes red, hot, broken, ulcerated and extremely painful

This condition can occur even though the temperature is well above freezing. Prevention is better than cure. Keep the feet dry and out of water and if possible wear rubber boots. If you do get water in your boots, take them off, empty them out and wring out the socks, replacing them as soon as possible. Check the feet frequently and rub them for five to ten minutes.

TREATMENT

Find a dry place to sit and remove one boot at a time. Gently dry the feet and wriggle your toes. Always allow the feet to warm up slowly and naturally, do not expose them to direct heat. If the skin has been broken, wash with clean water and gently apply an antiseptic cream. Elevate the legs to relieve any swelling and pain and do not walk until your feet have recovered. The best foot protection for walking over large areas of marshy ground are jungle boots which have a series of holes covered with mesh which let any water out.

Snow Glare/Blindness

Snow glare is a painful and watery inflammation of the eyeballs which causes a 'burning' sensation. When crossing snow on a bright sunny day, the eyes are exposed to

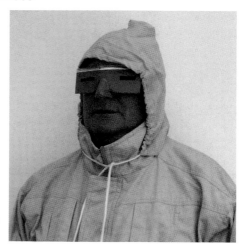

Improvised snow goggles

reflected rays diffused by snow particles that strike the eyeball from every direction. The first signs are of a gritty sensation in the eye, which can proceed to intense pain and loss of vision. Snow blindness can be distressing but it is not a serious condition. Prolonged exposure to ultra-violet rays of the sun pose the same hazards when travelling across the desert.

TREATMENT

Prevention is the best answer by protecting the eyes with sunglasses or snow goggles. If neither are available, a strip of cardboard, cloth or bark with narrow slits cut for eyes will suffice. Use charcoal from a cold campfire to blacken beneath the eyes to reduce glare.

Alcohol and Cold

Drinking alcohol while working in cold weather conditions is not a good idea. It will only serve to dilate the blood vessels and increase the amount of heat lost from the body. Additionally, winter activities such as skiing require an alert mind in order to prevent injury and avoid possible accidents.

HIGH ALTITUDE AREAS

Mountainous terrain can be divided into three zones – the lower slopes, the middle slopes and the high peaks – each of which presents their own problems. The lower slopes consist of the valley floor where flash flood and rivers can pose a potential risk. Fire and wild animals are a major danger on the middle slopes which are usually occupied by forest. The high peaks are normally solid slabs of rock and depending on the geographic location, the season will determine the

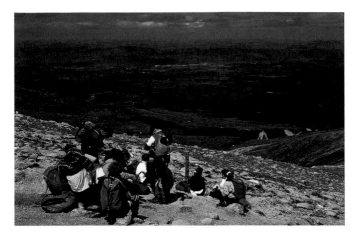

amount (if any) of snow covering and the possibility of avalanches.

Walking in the mountains at any time of year is a serious business, and in general, the higher you climb the higher the risk of accident or injury. Whether alone or in a group you should walk at a leisurely pace minimising physical effort. Walking too fast or lifting the legs over rocky or steep ground all put strain on the muscles and joints causing tiredness and aches. Arms and hands should be kept free, so that in the event of a slip or fall they can be used to fend off serious injury. Take extra care when climbing or descending steep slopes, and avoid scree areas: jumping over rocky terrain or running fast downhill is the easiest way to cause an injury.

If any form of serious rock climbing is required, the climber must be qualified enough to tackle the degree of severity that the rockface presents. Even where the rockface is easy, it is best to remember three basic rules:

➤ Avoid any loose rock when climbing and always make sure that you have three points of contact.

➤ Always make sure that it is possible to climb back down again if you need to.

➤ Stay out of snow fields, glaciers and overhanging snow.

Lightning Injury

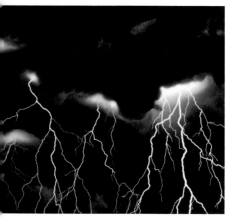

Lightning striking the ground normally seeks the easiest point to make contact – usually the highest point in the area – which is why it is wise to take precautions against it when in high mountainous regions. It is rare for an electrical storm to occur without some advance warning such as the appearance of thunderclouds in the distance followed by flashes of lightning and rumbles of thunder as the clouds approach. If lightning is anticipated, follow the precautions listed at the top of p. 165.

Lightning is almost always accompanied by rain and one should avoid both by finding shelter in a strong structure such as a cave or rock overhang. Staying dry

LIGHTNING PRECAUTIONS

➤ Stay away from peaks and high ridges

➤ Stay away from isolated trees or structures such as pylons, particularly if taller than the surrounding terrain

➤ Stay clear of tents (particularly those with metal poles) and metal equipment such as ice axes which would act as conductors

➤ Stay clear of others in your party, keeping 20-30 m (80-100 ft) between individuals

will prevent skin burn if you are unfortunate enough to be struck by lightning.

If caught out in the open by a lightning storm, with no chance of cover, sit down, preferably on your rucksack, and minimise your contact points with the ground as much as possible by drawing your knees up and placing your hands in your lap.

Whereas a domestic electrical injury travels through the body causing deep tissue damage and leaves a clear wound sign, lightning tends to travel outside the body. Such is the power of lightning that a direct strike will most often lead to death by cardiac arrest as the force disrupts all normal cardiac activity.

Those surviving a lightning strike will suffer from any or all of the symptoms outlined in the panel at the top of p.166.

LIGHTNING STRIKE SYMPTOMS

➤ Temporary paralysis is common

➤ Burns due to wet skin or metal jewellery

➤ Injury to the eyes and ears

➤ Fractured bones

➤ Memory loss

TREATMENT

Those struck by lightning must be treated quickly usually falling into three basic categories:

➤ Totally crisped (undeniably dead)

➤ Unconscious

➤ Conscious

Those that are unconscious should be attended to first. Lightning often causes the heart and respiration to stop and it is therefore vital perform your ABC regime (see p.22) as soon as possible. Those that are breathing should not be moved as lightning can easily fracture the neck and backbone (see p.100 on handling possible spine injuries). If CPR is necessary (see p.22) continue your efforts as long as it is physically possible, unlike other conditions such as heart attack.

Those that are conscious are going to be all right. They may be suffering from any of the above symptoms, all of which can be dealt with in order of priority. Treat any burns (see p.107), most of which will be on exposed or wet skin. However, in certain cases the lightning may cause a burn strip down the entire length of the body, which is not normally very deep. Check for individual puncture-type burns, which are normally a lot deeper but small enough in size to be treated without immediate hospitalisation.

Confusion and short-term memory loss are fairly common, and though conscious, the casualty may also suffer from temporary paralysis.

Acrophobia

Acrophobia is the fear of high places. Where a group of people have ventured into the mountainous wilderness, it can present a serious, even life-threatening problem. It is a fear that is resident in many 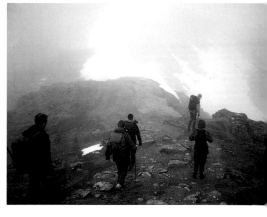 people but does not become apparent until they find themselves exposed at some height, such as on the side of a steep mountain. It is a normal part of the body's defence mechanism, and is sparked off in many cases by being confronted by the possibility of a fall.

The signs of acrophobia are gripping hold of strong points, with a reluctance to move up or down while the knees and lower leg may start to shake. On steep-sided mountains, especially where the party is roped together, this can pose a serious danger.

TREATMENT

Logic, reason and safety overcome momentary acrophobia in most people. If a person starts to shake with fear, they should be taken to solid ground and made to sit. An energy-rich drink often helps to calm the person. Where the party wish to continue, reason and additional safety devices may help sufferers overcome their fear. In extreme cases it is best to reassure the person and lead them to safety by retracing their original steps.

Altitude Sickness

This illness is caused by the reduction in atmospheric oxygen at altitudes above 2,400 m (8,000 ft), which leads to a reduction in the amount of oxygen in the blood and tissues. It usually arises in those who have not acclimatised to working at high altitudes or who have ascended too quickly to allow their body to

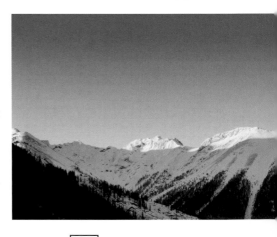

ALTITUDE SICKNESS SYMPTOMS

➤ Nausea and loss of appetite
➤ Persistent headache or light-headedness
➤ Fatigue
➤ Rapid heartbeat
➤ Breathing difficulties

cope with the atmospheric changes, although it can be very difficult to predict who will be affected and how severe the symptoms will be.

The symptoms of altitude sickness can appear within a few hours when working a height of around the 2,100 m (7,000 ft) or more.

The sickness becomes dangerous if allowed to persist, causing an increased intensity of the symptoms and the additional loss of balance and difficulty in walking.

TREATMENT

The priority with those suspected of altitude sickness is to rest and stop ascending. Fluid intake should be increased and asprin can be given to counter any of the symptoms. If these persist in spite of treatment, descend up to 900 m (3000 ft). Altitude sickness can be prevented by acclimatization prior to your excursion, although this can take several weeks. Where acclimatization has not taken place slowing the rate of ascent will help the body adjust.

If available, the drug acetazolamide can help prevent the symptoms of altitude sickness. Oxygen may be given as an emergency treatment but the only real cure is a slow descent to a safe altitude.

Dangerous Wildlife

The wilderness is far from being devoid of life. Most animals pose no threat but the dangers of predators, such as bears, are obvious while snakes if cornered will attack. On the other hand, some animals and insects will view you as a source of moisture and food. Insects likely to be a bother in this way are flies, lice and mites, which are not just unpleasant, but can also carry diseases such as dysentery and scrub typhus. Larger pests such as centipedes and some spiders may bite but are not necessarily fatal. On the other hand, invade the dwelling of certain scorpions and snakes and you may be inflicted with a bite that can cause death.

AUTHOR'S NOTE

➤ I have spent many years roaming the wilderness, from the northern tundra, across deserts and deep into darkened jungle and I can sadly validate that most animals are afraid of humans. Only when animals are hungry, disturbed in their local habitat, or wounded will they attempt to attack, even then, in the majority of cases it is in an effort to escape from humans.

BITES

Animal

The severity of bite damage will depend on the size and type of animal, with the majority of animal bites bring caused by either dogs or cats. Dog bites can inflict serious damage since a dog uses a body shaking movement when it bites which may tear the flesh and tendon. Furthermore, the bite of any large animal can exert sufficient pressure to crush bone, and deep penetration wounds are common.

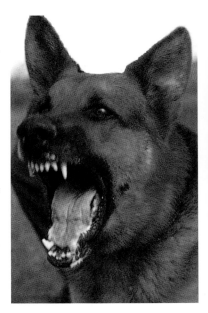

TREATMENT

Check to see if the casualty has a current tetanus inoculation (see p.70). Animal bites require vigorous cleansing (see p.72) with an antibacterial soap and the scrupulous removal of any debris. Debris should be suspected when the animal's teeth have penetrated an outer layer of clothing, such as a shirtsleeve, forcing foreign matter in the wound.

➤ Wash the wound three times a day using a solution of soap dissolved in water. This will help soothe the pain while removing any debris from the wound.

➤ Once the wound has been thoroughly cleaned, protect with a dressing and examine the wound on a daily basis.

➤ Check for bone damage and joint-space penetration.

➤ Where teeth have made deep puncture wounds that prove difficult to clean, the risk of secondary infection remains high. Check for signs of increased pain, discharge, swelling or red streaks around the wound site.

Animal bites rarely need closing and are best left open to assist drainage.

Rabies

Rabies can be carried by any mammal and is found in most countries, except the UK, Ireland and New Zealand; the problem is most marked in Asia, Africa and Central and South America. Although most people think of dogs when rabies is mentioned, wild animals such as foxes, skunks and bats can also carry the disease. It is rare for rodents or squirrels to be prone to

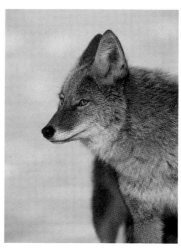

A wide range of mammals - other than dogs - pose a rabies threat

rabies but it is best to be very wary of any wild animal. A bite or even a lick from an infected animal transmits the disease, but it will need broken skin or a scratch to get into the bloodstream.

The early symptoms include headache, malaise, fever, loss of appetite, nausea, sore throat and a tingling sensation at the wound site. In the later stages the casualty becomes restless and agitated with escalating muscular spasms. There is also increased sensitivity to light, noise and touch and the common fear of water. The incubation period between infection and the onset of symptoms is anywhere from 30 to 60 days. Once the secondary symptoms appear, death is almost inevitable.

TREATMENT

If a suspect rabid animal bites you, you must seek post-prophylactic quickly. Rabies vaccines are usually successful but are most effective when administered as soon as possible after the incident. If you are planning to travel to an area where rabies is endemic, it may be wise to consider an anti-rabies vaccine before you leave.

In humans the virus is unstable and may even be washed out of a cut with copious amounts of soap and water if done immediately. If possible, the suspect animal should be killed or captured and handed over to a local health agency in order that the disease may be confirmed; this should only be considered where the animal is wild and there is no danger of further bites occurring as a result.

Human

It is rare that humans bite other humans but when they do it can be highly dangerous. Fights are a common cause for human bites and as such they are more prevalent with men as opposed to women. Common areas to be attacked are ears, nose, breasts, forearm and hands. In general humans do not inflict the same damage as one would expect to see from an animal bite. The problems arise from the risk of secondary infection caused by bacteria. Such infections cause serious illness that can be difficult to treat. Do not be concerned about contracting rabies from human bites.

TREATMENT

Treatment for human bites is the same as for animal bites. Where a human bite has been inflicted, it is vital to check that the patient's tetanus vaccinations are up to date (see p.70). The wound should be carefully cleaned with an antibacterial soap and irrigated with sterile water. When the teeth have penetrated an outer layer of clothing, such as a shirtsleeve, check for the presence of any foreign matter in the wound. Pay close attention to the wound checking for signs of increased pain, discharge, swelling or red streaks around the wound site. Human bites rarely need closing and are best left open to assist drainage, while applying normal wound care (see p.72). Suturing maybe required when flesh has been partly severed – this is common with bites to the ears or nose and a course of antibiotics should be started as soon as possible to reduce the risk of infection.

INSECT BITES AND STINGS

Insect bites, apart from being irritating, can leave the skin open to infection. Some insects also transmit diseases. It is important to be aware of the dangers and to take advantage of the several lines of defence that are available. Where the problem is extreme, cover your body with clothing as this reduces the amount of skin open to attack. Slow-burning, smoky fires will drive insects away, and it is best to light one on the windward side of camp. Place a ring of ash around your sleeping area or campsite to deter most crawling insects.

Lice

Human lice vary in length from 2–5 mm and are a flat wingless insect. The lice, of which there are three varieties – head, body and pubic – are transmitted mainly by person-to-person contact, 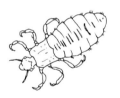 clothing and bedding. They have a lifespan of around four weeks but they reproduce quickly. Their main irritation is itching, which when a person is heavily infected can be quite maddening. More importantly, human lice can transmit typhus (see p.133), though such infections are rare.

Head lice can be seen crawling about the head. They breed rapidly and the females fix their eggs to the hair by means of a cement. These can be seen as small white oval-shaped bodies attached to the hair at intervals and are known as nits. The bite of the insect often causes itching which leads to scratching and subsequent infection of the skin by other organisms. The body louse lays its eggs both on the undercloth-ing and on the hairs of the body. As with head lice, the accompanying irritation causes scratching. Infection is generally through body contact or sleep-ing in unhygienic conditions. The pubic louse or crab is shorter and broader than the body or head louse. The crabs are transmitted mainly through sexual con-tact and burrow themselves into the skin around the pubis. They also cause itching.

TREATMENT

Both head lice and the nits (eggs) must be destroyed. Those medics in attendance should protect them-selves from infestation. An anti-parasitic shampoo, or lotion should be used for all three types of lice. One or two applications is normally enough to kill both lice and eggs. All infected clothing, sleeping bags, hats and hair brushes should be sterilized, or destroyed by burning.

Fleas

Fleas are carriers of plague and typhus.. To avoid catching them, stay away from any camels, dogs, cats or rats. It is not uncom-mon to come across the ruins of an ancient civilisa-tion in places such as the deserts of the Middle East. These are often used as resting places for nomadic tribes, and consequently they are infested with lice and fleas.

Mites

Mites are parasites, the female of which burrows into the skin, particularly on the front of the wrist, around the buttocks, the genitals and the feet and lays her eggs in the small tunnels she makes. This burrowing causes irritation, followed by scratching especially at night when the person is warm in bed. Extensive scratching can lead to secondary infection producing impetigo. The skin disease is spread by close contact with infected persons.

TREATMENT

There are various effective applications with which to treat this condition, including anti-parasitic creams or lotions. Treatment will only be successful if those in close contact with infected persons also receive treatment collectively.

Mosquitoes

Mosquitoes are found in most regions of the world, including the Arctic and temperate regions where they are not generally dangerous but constitute an irritating presence. While summer in the Arctic may seem fairly easy-going to the traveller it also brings a number of problems. The ground gets very soggy as

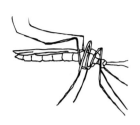

the snow melts which also announces the onslaught of biting insects. While small in size these insects can literally drive you crazy, making life unbearable. A good insect repellent in addition to covering the whole body and protecting the head with a net is the only real answer (see also Malaria, p. 000).

Flies

Flies are a bothersome pest in arid areas, especially around areas of moisture, which includes humans. Flies also ill carry disease and can cause infection of any small wound or cut. Sandflies are small black flies usually found in the subtropics. They are carriers of sandfly fever, which is a disease that is more unpleasant than

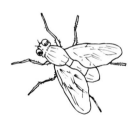

dangerous. The condition needs to be treated with rest and plenty of fluids. Ordinary netting will not keep out sandflies because they are so small, but they may be deterred by insect repellent. However, it is worth noting that these flies stay fairly low to the ground, flying up no more than 3 metres (10 ft). They also dislike moving air. To protect against flies, use the same measures as you would against mosquitoes. Also, make sure that any food supplies are not exposed.

Ticks

Ticks are crawling creatures measuring between 2 mm and 1 cm. They are bloodsuckers and possess strong piercing jaws.
Many tick bites are harmless but they are capable of transmitting a variety of serious diseases. There are two families of ticks which are able to transmit disease to humans. Soft 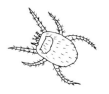 ticks hide in dilapidated buildings where there is poor hygiene. They usually are active at night and bite sleeping people. Hard ticks normally feed on animals, e.g. dogs, goats, rats, sheep, cattle, onto which they climb from the ground or vegetation. They can transmit tick typhus from animals to humans.

Avoiding Ticks

Preventing ticks from attaching themselves to you is the best way of avoiding tick-transmitted disease. Unless it is an emergency, you should not sleep in old buildings which have housed livestock. If you are camping out, ensure that the vegetation around the tent is kept short. Hard ticks are the most common but any disease will not be transferred if the tick is removed within 24 hours. Most DEET insect repellents are very effective against ticks. Check all over for ticks if you have been in an infested area.

TREATMENT

The first priority is to carefully remove the insect from the skin. The most effective way of doing this is to grasp the skin area around the tick's body with a pair of fine-point tweezers, and remove the tick with a sharp backwards pull. This does not hurt and is a far safer method than trying to induce the tick to disengage itself by any other method; burning the tick or applying chemicals will only force the tick to vomit, and crushing it will cause germs to enter the victim. If the head remains buried in the skin, remove it using the sterilised point of a needle. Treat localised pain with an ice pack.

Scorpions

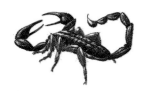

Scorpions are common and are easily recognised by their crab-like shape and high, forward curving tail with a stinger barb on the end. Their size varies from 1 inch (2.5 cm) up to 8 inches (20 cm). Their colour may vary too. They like damp, cool environments and tend to come out at night to hunt. They have a great tendency to hide themselves in discarded clothing, bedding and shoes. The majority of scorpion stings are not likely to cause death in a healthy adult. However, they are extremely painful and precautions should be taken to avoid them. If one of these creatures is crawling on you, knock it away in the direction it is moving, as most scorpions, despite

the speed of their stings, are unable to retaliate
quickly.

Spiders

Most spiders across the globe, in spite of occasionally
fiercesome appearances, do not cause major problems for travellers. However, there are a number
found in the Tropics, Australia, the Americas and the
Middle East whose bite can produce severe reactions
and on occasions, death. These species are illustrated
below.

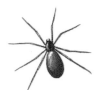

*Recluse or Fiddleback spider
(N. America) - identified by
the dark violin shape on the
back of the head*

*Black Widow or Hourglass spider
(common in warmer climates
across the globe) - identified by
the red, yellow or white markings
on the abdomen which are hour-
glass-shaped on some species*

*Funnelweb spiders
(Australia)*

Tarantula (Tropical Americas)

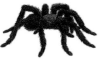

GENERAL SPIDER-BITE SYMPTOMS

Symptoms will vary depending on the particular species involved but in general all or some of the following will be in evidence

➤ Occasionally faint bite marks (sometimes appearing subsequently)

➤ Fever or chills

➤ Vomiting and nausea

➤ Joint pain

➤ Muscle stiffness or cramps

➤ Localised pain which can be severe

➤ A rash, discolouration or blister around the bite site

TREATMENT

The bite site should be cleaned thoroughly with soap and water. An ice pack on the site will also relieve pain. Pain relief medication can also be taken. If possible, the spider should be caught (dead or alive) to help identification. Evacuate to a medical facility as soon as possible.

Snakes and Lizards

Many reptile species are denizens of the desert, especially lizards and snakes. Most lizards can be disregarded as any sort of problem for, apart from a couple of exceptions in North America and Saudi Arabia, they are harmless. Snakes also thrive in the arid conditions and range from the completely innocuous to the deadly poisonous. Snakes tend to go for shady places such as under rocks, bushes and trees, so be wary when approaching such locations if venomous species are known to inhabit the area. Similarly, discarded clothing, bedding and boots should also be checked thoroughly before being put on. A selection of the most venomous snakes in different areas of the world is shown opposite.

TREATMENT

If you, or any other traveller suffers a snakebite your reaction must be rapid but without panic. The two major aims of snakebite treatment are to reduce the amount of venom entering the body, keeping it below a non-fatal dose if possible and to reduce the speed with which any venom circulates through the system, so that the body's own defence mechanisms can deal with it as it is absorbed.

➤ Any form of fear or panic – especially if violent exertion is involved – will instantly increase the rate of the heartbeat, and therefore the speed of the circulating blood. It cannot be too strongly stressed that rest and reassurance are high on the list of priority actions.

➤ While this is being given, the puncture site should be located and copiously washed with water.

➤ Do not cut the wound in any way, as this will merely open further channels through which venom can enter the bloodstream.

North abnd South America

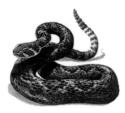

Rattlesnake

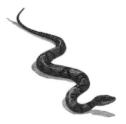

Copperhead

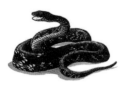

Cottonmouth or
Water Mocassin

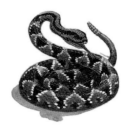

Tropical Rattlesnake

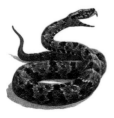

Fer de lance

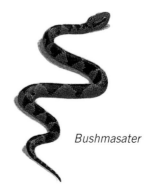

Bushmasater

Europe

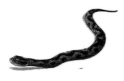

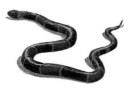

Adder

Coral snake

Africa & Asia

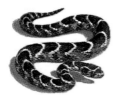

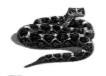

Scale-jawed viper

Puff adder

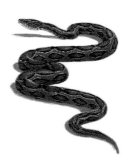

Russell's Viper

*Malay Pit Viper
or Mocassin*

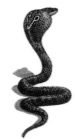

Cobra

Mamba

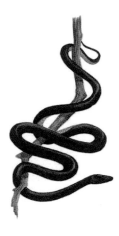

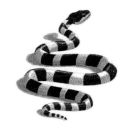

Krait

Boomslang

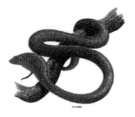

Australasia

*Australian
Brown Snake*

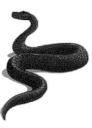

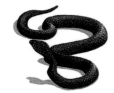

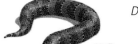

Death Adder

Australian Black Snake

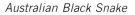

Tiger Snake

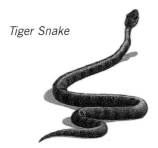

➤ Do not attempt to suck the venom out of the wound, because the lining of the mouth is able to absorb many substances with ease.

➤ Use a restrictive bandage. Apply it from above the bite, wrapping it downwards towards the puncture site. It should be applied tightly enough to stop the return of venous blood, since this is what will carry the venom into and around the body. But it must not stop the arterial blood supply to the area. The correct tightness of the restrictive bandage can be checked ensuring that, (a) there is still a feeble pulse below the bandage, and (b) that the veins below the bandage are distended. The bite will bleed after the bandage has been applied, but this is no cause for alarm. The escaping blood will very probably carry out with it some of the venom from the wound.

➤ The next step is to make sure that the bite site is as low as possible relative to the rest of the body. If practicable, put a splint on the limb. Immobilising it will lessen the possibility of any muscle movement having a pump-like action on the veins.

➤ Then immerse the bite in water – the colder the better – which will further slow down the return of blood.

➤ Reassurance should be constantly given, and the fear of death dispelled as far as possible. It will also lower the risk and therefore the seriousness of shock. If 15 minutes pass and there is no pain or swelling of the bitten area, and no headache or dryness of the mouth, then the bite was not poisonous.

Wild Animals

Attacks by animals smaller than a rabbit are rare, but larger animals can inflict serious wounding and infection. Most wild animals, even predators are 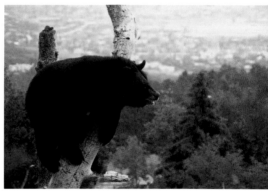 shy and are not often seen. Unless cornered, startled at close quarters or injured, they will seek to escape. Females with young are also likely to be protective and will attack anything perceived as a threat to their young. Large cats, such as lions, tigers, leopards and jaguar will sometimes attack a human if they look vulnerable or weak, or if that animal has tasted human flesh before. Far more dangerous are animals such as the hippopotamus, which accounts for more human deaths in Africa than any other animal, or even the

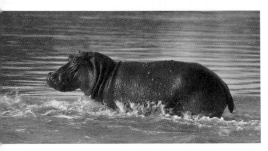

One of the major killers in Africa

water buffalo of Southeast Asia. These are not meat-eaters but can be extremely aggressive when roused or when feeling threatened. Elephants, too, should not be provoked, and should be given way to at all times. Unless there is reason not to, make as much noise as possible when passing through the jungle. This will act as a warning for many animals who will simply avoid you. The risk from animals and insects will depend largely on which continent and environment you are travelling through (for treatment see Animal Bites, p.172).

Evacuation & Rescue

With the respiration and circulation of a casualty stabilised and any blood loss stemmed, your next priority
should be to arrange evacuation to a proper medical
facility. The quicker this can be achieved the greater
are the chances of patient recovery.

If the group has been properly organised, then rescue
should be a matter of procedure rather than chance
or good fortune. Good communications, either by
word of mouth, radio, telephone or prearranged
schedule makes all the difference in a medical emergency. For many casualties the time elapse from the
moment the injury or illness occurs to that of reaching a proper medical facility can be vital to saving life.
This time lapse can be drastically shortened through
good communications.

When communications are not available the alternative is either to sit and wait for search and rescue to
find you, or to walk out. Neither of these options
stands the casualty in good stead. In the first instance
search and rescue teams must be aware that you have
a problem and then proceed to find you, which can
take from days to weeks to achieve. If you decide to
walk out, then you must consider how you are going
to carry the casualty. Remembering that in the wild

you may be forced to walk down narrow mountain tracks, or cross raging rivers. Even with four people carrying a stretcher it can prove an arduous and dangerous activity. Various factors will govern your final decision, such as the casualty's condition and their reaction to being moved, where the nearest help is, and how much time you have.

COMMUNICATIONS

There are many devices used for contacting and locating those who have become lost, and most provide similar functions and operations.

SARBE

One example is the SARBE 6 (*Search And Rescue BEacon*) which is designed for use as a survival radio by civil or military aircrew. On activation, the unit transmits a continuous, internationally recognised, swept-tone radio distress signal in the UHF243 Mhz 7.5kHz or VHF 121.5 Mhz 3,75 kHz distress frequencies. It also provides two-way voice communications between those needing help and the approaching rescuers. Built-in self-test facilities allow a simple confidence check to be carried out for correct functioning of the unit and battery state.

The unit is activated by the removal of an operating pin, either manually, by a single action, or automatically, by such functions as liferaft inflation or ejector seat operation. Simultaneous, omnidirectional transmission of both VHF and UHF signals then continues automatically for a minimum of 24 hours to facilitate detection by search aircraft or vessels, or by any other land, sea or airborne installation monitoring these frequencies. Pressel switches conveniently located on the side of the unit allow the user to select the voice mode, permitting two-way communication with the rescuers. Voice communication is on both distress frequencies simultaneously, and this mode is intended for use only when the operator can see or hear the rescue craft. The SARBE 6 is waterproof to a depth of 10 metres (32 feet).

Phones

Although mainly restricted to land usage, the global telephone network is extensive and accessible in many remote places. It is always worth taking a mobile phone with you for use in an emergency. There have been many successful rescues both in America and Great Britain through the use of mobile phones. Larger parties should consider carrying a portable satellite phone which are little larger than a laptop computer and will operate in every environment.

Global Positioning System (GPS)

The development of the Global Positioning System (GPS), which consists of 24 military satellites, has greatly increased the accuracy with which travellers can identify their position in the wilderness. Many outdoor enthusiasts now carry small hand-held GPS units which are no larger than a mobile phone. The GPS unit is able to receive and assimilate information from the satellites, converting it into a recognisable position and altitude at any point on the Earth's surface. The system is able to update your position as you move, recording speed and track in the process. It

GPS unit

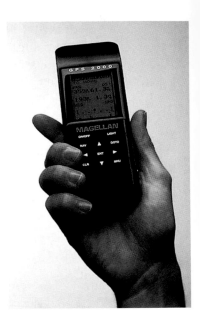

also allows you to pinpoint past and future waypoints, thereby taking away the need for recognisable landmarks. In a medical emergency the GPS will not only give you your present position to within a few metres, it will also allow you to accurately go forward or retrace your steps to the last known location where help can be summoned.

ASSESSING EVACUATION NEEDS

It is essential you consider all the factors when requesting an evacuation. These include the nature of the wound or illness, the type of evacuation transport available, and the nearness of medical facilities capable of dealing with the casualty. In many cases this decision is taken away from you once the casualty has been passed onto the rescue crew who will have a better knowledge of the medical services available. You should also remember that rescue efforts are costly and in some countries may require payment. The need to evacuate must therefore be balanced against the casualty's survivability.

It is therefore down to the medic to assess the need

and type of evacuation. For example, those casualties in immediate danger, such as survivors of a heart attack, severe body mass loss, internal bleeding and shock, will require urgent evacuation. On the other hand, casualties suffering from a broken leg, burns, malaria or dysentery, but who in the opinion of the medic require evacuation from the wilderness, will only require a non-priority evacuation.

TRAVELLING

Without communications, it is difficult to assess whether there will be a rescue attempt, and even if there is, it would be presumptive to believe that they will locate you quickly if in a vast wilderness. To travel or stay put is one of the great dilemmas when confronted with any serious medical emergency in the wilderness. Even if the casualty can be moved, you must possess the physical ability and resources to carry them.

Walking Out

Once you have determined the need to travel, you must prepare. Before you start, it is important to check the weather and work out a travel routine based on the type of terrain and conditions you'll be passing through.

Unless you have good reason to believe that help is closer by pressing on with your journey, it is always best to retrace your steps (see GPS, p.193). This has two main advantages: your knowledge of the terrain and a known time factor until you reach help. If a situation has arisen whereby your present position and that of the nearest help is unknown to you, then you should look for populated areas or lines of communication (see below) to head for. Unfortunately, most centres of population and lines of communications run in the lowlands, so if you are stuck with a casualty in the mountains, you must first descend. The route of your decent should be based on the easiest way down which leads towards any known or visible populated area. If you are not sure where this is, walk downhill until you find a water course, as almost all human habitats are to be found on or near a river. Once on the move, the pace should be steady and unrushed with a break of 5–10 minutes at least every hour. Use this break productively to check on the casualty and to consider how the travel is affecting them. Use the rest stops to change over those personnel who are carrying the casualty. Make sure that no one exceeds their physical limits.

Lines of Communication

It is rare to find a road in an isolated area but there are some, usually in order to service a commercial enterprise. Other artificial features likely to be found in remote areas are oil pipelines, wells, refineries, crushing plants, military

installations and telecommunications equipment. Power lines are a particularly good feature to follow because they always lead to civilization and normally have a clear access through forest and over rocky terrain. However, where such man-made features do not exist your best bet is to follow a watercourse.

Local Populations

Meeting with the local population is likely to mean that help will be within reach. However, you may be in a remote area of a foreign country where you are the stranger, so be aware and respectful of local laws and customs.
Unfortunately, many travellers have found themselves imprisoned for unknowingly breaking a law. It is also not that uncommon for 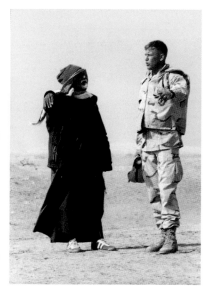 travellers to be held hostage for ransom in the more troubled parts of the world.

But it is more likely that meeting the local people should see an end of your problems. In many cases, even isolated peoples will have some form of communication with the outside world. If not, at least they will have food, water and shelter, and probably have better modes of transport. They will also know where the nearest help can be found and perhaps help with carrying the casualty. In the event of such an encounter, there are a number of basic rules to observe.

➤ Unless you are literally dying, wait outside their village until welcomed.

➤ Spread your palms to show you are unarmed before shaking hands.

➤ Take any drink or food that is offered, and remember to thank your host.

➤ Treat all people, customs and religion with respect.

➤ Explain your situation, use simple drawing in the dirt.

➤ Talk to the men, and do not openly approach or talk to the women.

➤ Other than for medical reasons, do not remove your clothes in public.

➤ Explain that you must move on as soon as possible.

➤ Thank them for their kindness when you leave.

Carrying an Injured Person

A moderately injured or ill person who still has all or partial leg function should be assisted between two helpers. For a casualty who needs to be carried the method will depend on the number of people available. One-on-one carry techniques, such a the fireman's lift) and piggyback (oppositet), are only possible for a very short distance. In most cases, a stretch-

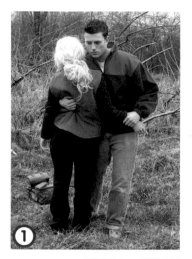

(1)

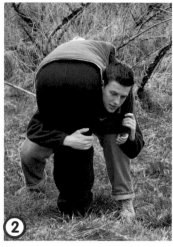

(2)

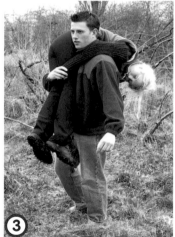

(3)

Pictures 1–3 show the technique for a fireman's lift

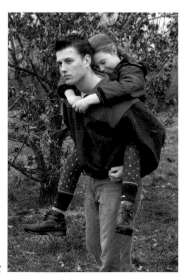

Piggyback

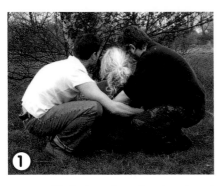

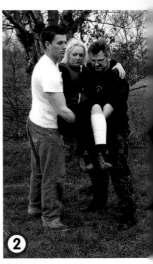

Technique for a two-hand seat

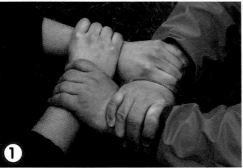

Technique for a four-hand seat

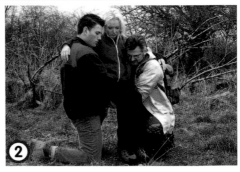

Crutch-carry technique

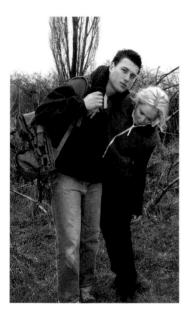

er, even an improvised one, should be used. A makeshift stretcher can be improvised by threading two jackets onto poles, with a belt to give it a bit more stability at the middle. If you have to lift a patient to get them on a stretcher, make sure that the body is kept in line and that each part is well supported; in particular, ensure that the centre of the stretcher isn't sagging. If a patient has suspected spinal injuries, do not attempt to move them (see p.100).

Movement in the Dark

There maybe times when a casualty is so ill that you need to move them in the dark; likewise, there are certain terrain such as the desert where it is beneficial to move during the night. If, for whatever reason, moving in darkness is the only option in your situation, you need to do this safely. Being in complete darkness can be frightening, so stay calm and take stock of your situation. Check that you have no other source of lighting on you. If you are moving with other people, make sure that everyone stays within touching distance with the next person. If you have a rope or lifeline, rope everyone together, placing the weakest in the centre.

Unless a life really depends on it, do not try crossing a river in darkness – it is extremely dangerous. Likewise, though it is a good idea to follow a stream or river on the flat, never follow water down a steep mountainside, as it will inevitably have a waterfall somewhere. Even if the waterfall is small, it will be enough to cause injuries if you fall over in the dark.

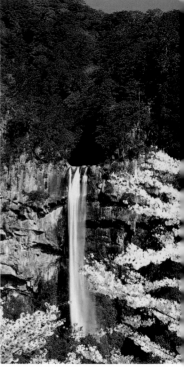

Working in complete darkness produces what is known as night sight, a condition where the eyes adjust to the low level of available light. This will be interrupted if a torch or naked flame is used, so always close one eye against bright lights. All the human senses become heightened when enveloped in darkness, and these should be used to their best advantage. However, be aware that heightened senses mean even familiar noises may sound much louder and closer, which to some people can be unnerving – stay calm, and talk to yourself or each other if necessary.

Prior to darkness falling, check the ground you

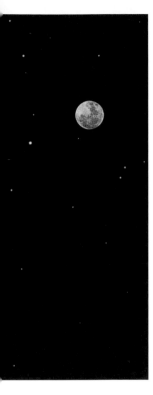

intend to cross and memorise your route. If your memory is good, it will help you to keep to your route during the darkness. Your sense of distance can become confused, as you will be moving more slowly than you think. Try, if possible, to locate features which can be easily identified. Touch is particularly helpful when it is totally dark or when you are moving over steep and rocky ground. Again, always move downhill, using your hands as if you were a climber, keeping three points in contact with the rock at all times. Use your hands and arms to make sure that the immediate space before you is clear of any obstacles and is secure to step on. If the ground is uneven or there is the possibility of a dangerous drop, crawl on your hands and knees. Stop when you hear water, as this almost certainly indicates a drop of some height. Try throwing a stone and listen for the sound of it hitting earth or water, as this should indicate distance and depth.

Light contrast is a good aid to night navigation. Snow-covered ground reflects any starlight and moonlight, but be aware that it also hides pitfalls below the surface. On a clear moonlit night it is possible to see for

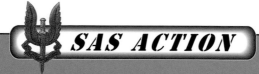

up to 100 metres over open terrain. Walking in a forest at night generally means there is little or no light. Stretching the arms out in front of the body will warn of low branches. There is also a contrast between the dark forest and the lighter sky, which can act as guide if a track is being followed through a forest. Simply look up and observe the treetop silhouette. Certain weather conditions provide a fair amount of lightning which will constantly illuminate the surrounding area, albeit briefly.

River Crossing

Sometimes when confronted with a major river there is little option other than to cross it. The width of the river, its depth and strength of current all pose problems, as does the type of riverbed. Mud and silt can be extremely dangerous, to the point where you become permanently stuck or worse, sucked below the surface. Few riverbeds are flat and most have hidden depths into which anyone crossing may fall. Strong currents can dash the best of swimmers into

RIVER CROSSING

➤ Plan your route to avoid having to cross water

➤ Always look for the safest crossing place

➤ Cross only if absolutely necessary

➤ Choose the widest and shallowest stretch

➤ Never, unless the alternative is life-threatening, attempt to cross a river in flood

➤ If alone, use a buoyancy aid

➤ Use a safety line if available

rocky outcrops, or plunge them into falling rapids. All these obstacles must be taken into account before attempting to ford any river. Never cross on a river bend as the speed of the current and the depth of the water will increase from the inside of the bend to the outside. Instead, choose a wide stretch where the water is flowing more slowly. Avoid any temptation to jump from stone to stone as these are often slippery and a fall could result in a sprain or a fracture, plus you may drop vital equipment.

If you flounder or slip in the water and find yourself floating downstream, it is important not to panic. Float feet first going with the current, fend off any obstacles until you feel the riverbed below you and are able to stand, or you have reached the safety of the riverbank. Depending on the weather conditions, you are advised to remove your socks and trousers before wading any river. This will provide you with

immediate comfort and
warmth when you reach
the opposite bank.

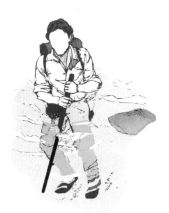

When crossing a river
alone use a stout stick to
provide extra stability in
the water and for testing
the depth of the riverbed,
potholes and underwater
obstacles (see right).

If a rope or line is at hand
and you are with a companion, make sure that the
person crossing is safely secured to the bank. Or
follow the procedure illustrated below, which will
always ensure that the person crossing is assisted by at
least two others.

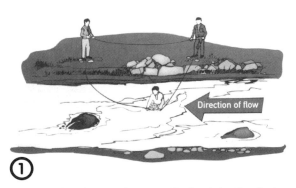

*The rope is taken to the opposite bank by the first -
person, who should be the strongest swimmer; he should
be secured to the safety so that he can be pulled back if
he gets into difficulties.*

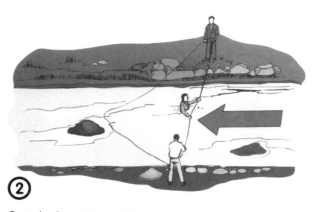

② Once he is across and the line is secure, the next member and each of the rest of the party should secure themselves to the line and pull themselves across.

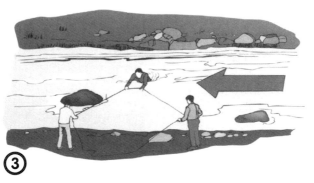

③ The last member of the party should attach himself to the line and be pulled across. If possible, weaker swimmers should have the benefit of a second line to aid and secure them.

If the water is too deep for wading and you have to swim across, make a buoyancy aid. Your rucksack secured in an airtight survival bag will make an excellent aid – these can be joined if the party consists of three or four people.

All those suffering illness or injury should be assisted by linking arms around each others shoulders, with the weakest swimmer in the middle. Move across the river with the strongest member against the flow of the current, moving slowly and supporting each other if one should stumble or fall. Take care when entering and leaving the stream especially if the banks are steep. Hold onto the bank and help the weakest person out first. If the river is too deep for wading, place the injured party on top of a secured bouncy aid such as several rucksacks lashed together.

Rafts

Rivers and their immediate surrounds contain many resources useful in a wilderness medical emergency. In the jungle, rivers offer a swift and excellent transit route. A raft will transport a sick or injured person with little or no buffeting. However, it is important that the condition of the river be assessed before using a raft as not all

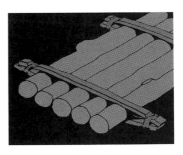

A simple raft construction: gripper bars, notched at the end to provide a better hold for the ropes, are secured over wooden spars. Additional buoyancy could be added beneath the spars

rivers are flat and calm. Upturning your raft in a deep and fast running river will do little to improve the condition of your casualty.

Forget any ideas about constructing a canoe or any other complex construction: this takes skill and a great deal of time, and requires specialist bits such as resin for waterproofing. However, making a raft is within everyone's capabilities. Rafts can be built with anything that has a degree of buoyancy – empty bottles wrapped in a polythene bag, old oil drums or wood. If using wood, try to use the lightest available. Once your raft has been constructed, ensure that all your supplies and equipment are firmly secured, in case it tips over. Do not attach too much stuff to your person because the weight may prevent you from staying afloat if you fall in.

To steer your craft around obstacles in the river, such as rocks or rapids, use a long punting pole (see illustration, right). If your journey takes several days, take care to securely moor your raft at each campsite. Check the raft for service-ability every morning and repair as required.

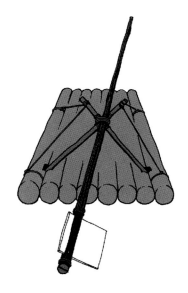

Constructing a Raft

A raft is basically anything that floats with enough buoyancy to support a human being. The secret behind any good raft is its strength and durability. The materials for making a raft can vary from brush-wood and logs to polythene sacks and ponchos. Their construction needs little imagination and several ideas are highlighted below. Keep in mind that it is trapped air which makes a raft float.

WAITING TO BE RESCUED

If you have communications or the casualty cannot be move, then your best bet is to sit tight. Search and rescue (SAR) contingency plans will come into operation at the first sign of trouble, either when a radio distress call is received, or if prearranged waypoint call-in procedures have been missed.

If for any reason your location is not known, then SAR teams will be called in to make a search. The area covered will be based on the best estimated overall guide of the last known location. How the search is carried out will be determined by the size of the area to be covered, the terrain, the weather and operational necessity. If radio communications can be established, or a beacon signal is received, then a contact search will be initiated. This is designed to concentrate rescue efforts on a relatively small area, thus increasing the speed in which rescuers can get to you.

Unless there is accurate knowledge of the location of the party to be rescued, it will be futile and even risky to send out search teams during the night. In the event, a search plan will be devised, and search patterns allocated to the aircraft.

Search patterns

There are three main types of search pattern:

➤ Area search. This involves dividing up the area into smaller areas, using natural features and landmarks as boundaries in which individual teams are to search.

➤ Sweep search. The rescue party will spread out in a line and search the area in a disciplined and organised manner.

➤ Contact search. A search focused on a smaller area but based on the principles of the sweep search.

SIGNALLING RESCUERS

If you are stranded with a medical emergency and awaiting rescue, then you should prepare some form of emergency signal in order to attract attention. Such action can greatly reduce the amount of time it takes for any search party to locate you.

Signalling is a means of localized communication which can take the form of shape, sound, silhouette and sight. Sound can encompass anything from shouting, to blowing a whistle, while sight can mean using a signalling mirror or making a smoking fire. Whichever signalling method you choose will depend on what equipment is available and the conditions you find yourself in.

Light

Light is the ideal signal attraction at night and it can be emitted from any number of sources such as a fire, torch, strobe, camera or flare.

Although extremely effective, the problem with most flares and torches is that they are either limited to one single usage or for the duration of the batteries. All emergency flares come with operating and safety instructions so make sure you read them before setting off. Consider if small hand-held flares would be better used to light a larger signal fire.

Signal Fires

A signal fire needs to be prepared and ready to be lit at a moment's notice. Make sure they will ignite instantly by placing plenty of light, dry tinder in the middle. Your rescue may come at any time of night or day, so when the moment arrives remember you need

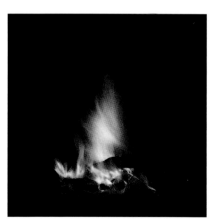

to produce contrast. By day you can produce white smoke by burning green or damp vegetation on top of a very hot fire. At night, a large bright fire gives the clearest signal. Be careful when siting your signal fire in order not to cause a forest fire.

Mirror & Heliograph

Any type of mirror (the larger the better) is excellent for signalling, providing you have bright sunshine. It is simply a matter of reflecting the sun's rays toward a search plane or party to attract their attention. All aircraft or vehicles carry a number of mirrors that will serve as a signalling device. A more accurate method is to use a purpose-made heliograph. Modern variations of these are smaller than a computer disk measuring just 5cm x 5cm (2 x 2 inches) yet they have the capacity to accurately reflect some 85 per cent of sunlight up to a range of some 20 km (12 miles). Mirrors work very well in the desert and areas where sunlight is guaranteed. Once any rescue aircraft has spotted you, stop signalling as you will only blind the pilot.

Flares

There are many different types of missile flare on the market. Some simply fire a glowing light which lasts a few seconds, and some have a parachute attached which will retard the flare's descent making it visible for longer. Always read the instructions carefully and follow them to the letter. For added safety always keep the flare pointing skywards. Parachute flares are one shot, so make sure their use is justified. Likewise, the number of normal flares with any pistol is usually a maximum of nine. Flares are particularly useful where there is dense overhead foliage obscuring you from the SAR aircraft.

Torches & Smoke

Any torch is a bonus at night, but for signalling, a

large broad beam is
required if any rescue
aircraft is to see it.
Moving the torch from
left to right in a slow
arch will help attract
attention, as will shining
it into a reflective sur-
face, because it is not the
light the search aircraft
sees but the movement
of light. Strobes are
designed to create this
effect by emitting an
extremely bright pulsat-

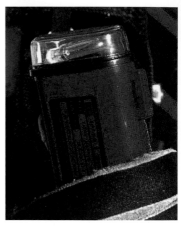

Rescue torch

ing light. On a clear night a strobe can be seen some
16 km (10 miles) away and is effective in all terrains.

A modern camera flash also makes a good signalling
device, but as with other battery-powered systems it
is limited in life and needs to be used sparingly. In
cold climates batteries are best kept warm to maintain their performance.

Balloons

Radar-reflective, and colour-detectable balloons
come in a variety of sizes. The coloured versions
were primarily designed for the jungle, where they
could be inflated and raised above the canopy. The
balloons, which are normally constructed of bright
orange polythene, are inflated by mixing chemicals
with water to produce helium gas. As the balloon
fills it is raised on a line and tethered where it can

be clearly seen by search aircraft.

Radar-reflective balloons are more compact, and are more automated in their operation. Inflation starts with the removal of a safety pin, and the activation of a helium cartridge that fills the balloon. The balloon is tethered to the life jacket from where it raises to around 100ft, where it will remain even in strong winds for up to five days.

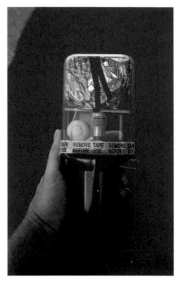

Radar-reflective balloon

The radar reflective signature has a 10m signature which can be detected by search vehicles up to 30 kilometres away. Balloons are excellent for signalling at sea.

Ground-to-Air Signals

The letters and configurations shown below are used in ground-to-air recognition signals. When constructing them take into account that a pilot may be a long way off and therefore the size and background colour contrast of the signal is extremely important. This can be done by making your signals at least 5 m (15 ft) long and about 1.5 m (5 ft) wide. Black earth against light-coloured grass, or shadow created by tramping down fresh snow or laying down fir branches, will all add to the contrast.

Ground-to-Air signals

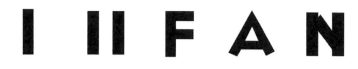

I	**II**	**F**	**A**	**N**
Require a doctor and Casevac	*Need medical supplies*	*Need food and water*	*Yes - affirmative*	*No*

△	**LL**	**X**	**→**	**□**
Safe to land	*Everything OK*	*Unable to move*	*Moving this way*	*Need compass and map*

The illustration opposite shows the code for ground-to-air body signallling.

HELICOPTER RESCUE PROCEDURES

Most SAR teams are organised along military lines and use either aircraft or helicopters. The latter has the added advantage of being able to land or hover. The SAR crews are highly skilled and have access to excellent resources. Most carry personnel and facilities for front-line medical care. However, it would be a dangerous mistake to assume that they will always be there to get you out of danger. For various reasons, such as the rescue team not knowing your location or serious weather conditions, the team is

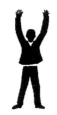

Pick us up

*Need
mechanical
help*

Land here

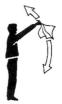

Yes

No

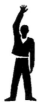

All is well

*Can proceed
shortly*

Have radio

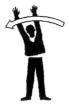

*Do NOT
attempt to
land here*

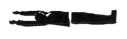

*Need medical
assistance*

*Use drop
message*

not always able to operate immediately. Even when your position has been located, helicopter crews can take a considerable amount of time assessing whether they can land or not. It is not uncommon over rough seas or jungle terrain for the pilot to make several attempts at establishing a hover close enough to the casualty to be able to get a winchman or mountain rescue team to their position.

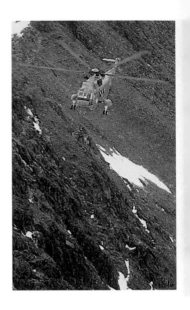

Having arrived at a workable hover, the next priority is to assess the safest method of rescuing the survivors. To ensure that no important aspect of the situation is overlooked, SAR crews use a standardised system of priorities which in descending order are:

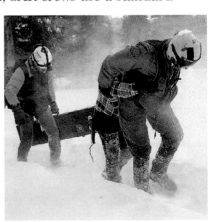

➤   Aircraft safety.

➤   Winchman safety.

➤   Casualty / survivor safety.

ESTABLISHING A LP

➤ First check that the surface will support a helicopter, for example, that the ground isn't waterlogged, there are no large rocks, fallen trees or pot holes.

➤ Next make sure that it is free of any debris or objects that would be blown about by the rotor downdraught.

➤ Check the approach path, which will be into the prevailing wind, to make sure there are no tall obstructions.

➤ Mark the centre of your LP with some form of marker, and indicate to the pilot the wind direction, improvising a wind sock or by making smoke (p. 000).

Landing Areas

Where possible the helicopter will land to evacuate a casualty; to make this a viable option, those on the ground should do everything to provide a good landing pad (LP). This involves several factors, such as size of possible landing area, ground slope, surface type and the direction of wind and approach.

Safety

Wait until the helicopter has landed and either the pilot or a crew member has clearly indicated to you to advance forward. Never approach a helicopter from the rear or by descending down a slope, as both will put you in extreme danger from the rotor blades. The best approach is on the cabin door side at a 45 degree angle from the helicopter nose.

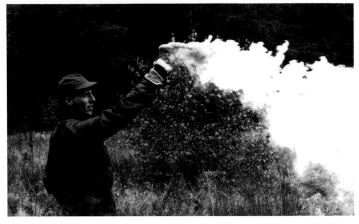

Smoke can be used to show the wind direction across the LP

Rescue Strops

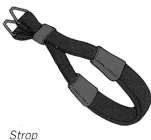

Strop

Where the rescue heli-copter is unable to land, they will lower a strop harness, or a winchman. The helicopter rescue strop is designed primarily to facilitate the rescue of survivors. It can be used at sea or on land to lift uninjured survivors of any size with relative ease. There is a 'D' ring at each end of the strop, the centre portion is cushioned with a rubber sheet comfort pad tapered at each end and covered with polyester fabric. A sliding toggle, through which the two ends of the of the strop pass, enables the wearer to draw the strop close to his body before the ascent. There is a webbing handle at the centre of the strop at the wearer's back, which enables the winchman to grasp the survivor and guide him back into the aircraft cabin.

Winching Techniques

Most helicopter rescues involve lowering a crew member to assist those being winched aboard, but in certain circumstances, this may not be feasible and so a one-man lift will be necessary. When the helicopter is positioned into the wind,

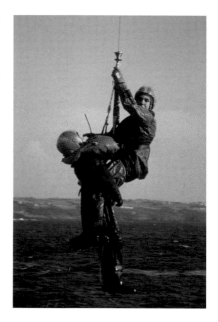

overhead the person to be rescued (who must be conscious and uninjured), a rescue strop will be lowered. The survivor places the strop over his head with the winch cable to the front. It should be adjusted under the armpits and tightened using the webbing-ring grommet, before signalling to the winch operator that he is ready. A more common method is a double lift which involves the lowering of a crewman from the helicopter to a survivor who will be secured with the strop and raised together with crewman. Similar methods are used at sea or on land, by day or night. Stretcher cases will always be supervised by a lowered crew member.

Travel Preparation & Planning

Any travel whether it be a package tour to Spain or a spontaneous walk through the Himalayas requires some planning and preparation.

Although all travellers are at risk from illness and injury, research has shown that those between the ages of 20 and 40 suffer most. This is primarily due to younger travellers being accompanied by their parents and who, along with the older traveller, are less likely to take risks. Age considerations also play a large part in the type of travel and location chosen. For example, you are unlikely to find a child or a pensioner taking part in potentially dangerous activities such as mountaineering, parachuting and white-water rafting. Additionally, the majority of people who prefer to go trekking into the wilderness or on budget holidays to isolated places fall into the 20- to 40-year-old age bracket. The risk differential derives not just from the remoteness of an area but also from the lack of suitable and available medical assistance.

We read more and more about one extremist group or another is holding more and more Western travellers captive. Those who travel into isolated areas, especially where insurrection and war are active, risk becoming a captive. While the cause of the terrorists may differ from political demands to poverty, the circumstances for the captives are usually the same. You will be held in squalid conditions, fed on poorly cooked food and possibly beaten. In such an environment, your body and health will quickly decline.

The greater the climatic and cultural contrast of a country, the greater the risk of danger. The extremes of heat, cold and wet almost all exist in isolated and unpopulated areas. These extremes also present a whole range of unforeseeable medical problems. Cultural problems can arise through differing political conditions, religious intolerance, war zones, isolated tribes and Third World deficiencies. Any of these can result in wounding, capture or death.

Diligent planning is essential to ensure that the trip is both pleasant and free from disasters. It is wise to follow established guidelines for visiting wilderness areas. These can seem over-fussy and restrictive but if adhered to, they could well save a life during an unforeseen emergency. Guidelines are even more vital when a group of young, or inexperienced people take to the wilderness with little or no knowledge of the culture or current political situation. In such a case, it is up to the party leader to be responsible for the implementation and strict adherence to certain safety procedures, albeit without losing the initial thrill of the adventure.

Once the location has been decided on, as much information as possible about the area needs to be gathered. Maps, guidebooks and local people can all provide valuable facts about good, interesting routes. In particular, make sure that the location is accessible at the time you are planning to go – floods, famine and natural disasters happen all the time.

Take into consideration the modes of transportation available in the chosen country and how you intend to enter the wilderness. Depending on the climate, consider your dress, footwear and any other essential equipment. If you are in a group, it is important that the group leader checks that each individual is properly prepared prior to setting off.

Finally, if you are planning a trip that is lengthy, is to a remote location or comprises a large number of people, make sure you can answer 'yes' to these three questions:

➤ Do you have and can you maintain communication?

➤ Is there a medically qualified person within your group?

➤ Do you have a good medical pack?

MEDICAL EXAMINATION

Before embarking on any long-term, strenuous activity, such as walking in the outback, you would be well advised to go to your doctor for a full medical check-up. Making sure that your body is in good shape and able to carry out the task you intend to set yourself is as equally important as taking along a good medical pack. If you are currently taking medication, make sure you have an adequate supply.

If your wilderness adventure includes lots of walking then a session with a chiropodist may save you hours of pain and misery caused by foot disorders and poor fitting shoes.

IMMUNISATION

Many diseases such as typhoid, paratyphoid, yellow fever, typhus, tetanus, cholera and hepatitis can all be vaccinated against. It is essential to obtain as many vaccinations as possible, making sure your immunisation records are kept up to date. Prior to visiting any foreign country you are advised to seek current medical advice and take extra immunisations and precautions. Make sure you carry a good supply of anti-malarial tablets where needed.

PERSONAL HYGIENE

Protection against illness starts with hygiene. Care in preparation of food and drink, proper waste disposal, and effective insect and rodent control will greatly reduce the risk of disease. If possible, wash daily with warm water and soap. A small amount of water can be used to sponge the face, armpits, crotch and feet at least once a day. Underclothing collects dirt and sweat so keep it dry and clean, especially if you are unable to change on a daily basis. If clothing cannot be washed it should be shaken vigorously and exposed to the sun and air at least once a day. The sun is a useful agent against disease, as few bacteria or viruses can survive exposure to ultraviolet light.

Parasitic infections are common the world over. In their ordinary state, they are little more than annoying; however, almost all such infections cause irritation which leads to scratching. Scratching normally breaks the skin and allows infection to develop. Good personal hygiene and avoidance are the best ways to avoid parasitic infection. Puncture wounds from bites can also cause skin infections.

Avoid scratching any rash. As a basic rule of thumb dry rashes should be kept damp by covering the area with a clean cloth compress; wet rashes should be kept dry. If no medical preparations are available, a concentrate of tannin made by boiling tree bark (left to cool) will help. A small rendering of boiled animal fat and crushed charcoal rubbed into a dry rash will help prevent the skin cracking and promote healing. Fungal infections are best exposed to direct sunlight whenever possible and kept dry. All skin rashes that become infected should be treated as open wounds and dressed accordingly.

DENTAL PROTECTION

We must eat and as a result small amounts of food and bacteria (plaque) become adhered to our teeth and gums. Our mouths can suffer a bacterial infection if this plaque is allowed to build up. This is prevented by brushing and flossing on a regular daily basis.

Unclean teeth run the risk of gingivitis, when the gums become red and swollen. One such indicator of this is when you are cleaning your teeth and spit out blood. If gingivitis is allowed to go unchecked, it can lead to a dental abscess, loosening of the tooth and eventually tooth loss. A tooth abscess in the wilderness can cause severe tooth pain and continuous discomfort.

The best treatment is prevention, which starts with a regular check-up prior to travelling. Brushing your teeth at least twice a day and rinsing with an antiseptic mouthwash will protect you teeth against infection. For those who have developed a tooth abscess while in the wilderness, painkillers and a course in oral antibiotics is recommended. Pain-relief medications will only help subdue the ache, the real solution is to combat the abscess.

In extreme situations an improvised toothbrush can made by chewing the end of a stick to separate the fibres; use a stick only once and then discard. Lye slurry, soap, sand and salt can all be used instead of toothpaste. The inner strands of paracord or the fine fibres on the inside of tree bark can be utilised as dental floss. A mouthwash can be made from salt water, or by boiling pine needles (allow to cool). Painful cavities can be filled with candle wax to help relieve the pain.

EYES

Visit your optician before travelling. You will not be going far if your eyesight is impaired. If you wear glasses, make sure you take at least one spare pair with you and likewise for contact lenses. In the wilderness if you can't see, you can't walk. Sunglasses are therefore a must in both bright sunlight and snowy conditions.

HAIR

Hair can attract lice and is best kept short. For any long-term travelling into a remote area (more than one week), all members of the party should have cropped hair.

Shaving should not be encouraged during cold weather as it leads to cracked skin. If facial problems arise, such as sores or boils, it is best not to shave at all.

FEET

Your feet are your personal transport, and without them, you are going nowhere. Walking and climbing over rough ground can take its toll on both your feet and boots, so make sure you keep both in good order. Sweat accumulates in the footwear and may accelerate rotting as well as create conditions for blisters and fungal diseases of the foot. At least once a day boots should be taken off and aired. Socks, too, will need to be dried or changed when they become wet. A small exposure (30 mins) to the late afternoon sun will help dry boots and socks, and help prevent any fungal diseases developing on the feet.

Blisters & Ingrown Toenails

Feet require constant maintenance and blisters or ingrown toenails can be extremely painful and prevent the traveller from walking. Foot blisters are usually caused by ill-fitting boots, poor quality socks or loose laces combined with long periods of having to walk over rough, uneven ground. Stop and treat small blisters immediately by covering them with surgical tape. A severe blister is often filled with fluid, and can be made more comfortable if the fluid is removed. Large blisters which look about to burst and rupture the skin should be punctured with a sterilised needle and thread. Run the needle through the blister leaving the threads hanging out, this will ensure that the fluid drains without creating a large break in the skin. Make sure that the surrounding area is kept thoroughly clean and dry.

Ingrown toenails should be treated as soon as they become apparent. As an emergency treatment, without removing the nail, the best method is by shaving the top centre of the nail with a scalpel blade from your medical kit. Skim the middle third of the nail shaving away from the bed towards the nail-tip. Place a thin piece of plastic under the nail to prevent accidentally cutting the toe front. When the nail is thin enough it will buckle into a ridge and relieve the outer pressure. Removing the nail altogether should be avoided, as this will require a dressing and may prevent the patient from walking for several days.

Medical Packs

It is absolutely vital that the first aid kit is tailored to the nature of the trip you are about to undertake. Your pack should reflect:

➤ The length of the trip

➤ The remoteness of the location and likely distance to the closest medical facility

➤ The number of members in the party

➤ The terrain to be covered and/or the likely activities to be undertaken

➤ The first aid or medical skills of your party

COMMERCIALLY PREPARED PACKS

It is best to avoid commercially prepared first aid packs unless they been specifically designed for serious outdoor. The Gregson Lifesaver System is one

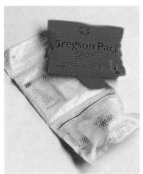

such pack. It has been designed to help perform first-aid procedures as you read aloud the instru-ctions, which saves vital seconds. The instructions are easy to follow and the contents easy to find, covering all eventualities from blisters to bleeding, fractures to burns, and even rescue.

CREATING YOUR OWN MEDICAL PACK

If you prefer to assemble your own personal medical first-aid kit, consider carefully what items you will include. The range of survival equipment is vast, with new items coming onto the market every year. However, there are several vital questions you should ask yourself about each item:

➤ Is it really necessary?

➤ Is its function duplicated by any other item?

➤ Are you capable of using the item?

Remember, the aim is to keep the kit as compact as possible. Once selected, assemble all the pieces of equipment you intend to carry and make sure they are well packed in a totally waterproof container, preferably one which is in a high-visibility colour. The simplest way of ensuring the pack is waterproof is to seal the whole kit in an airtight, plastic, snap-seal food container; individual items within the pack can also be sealed in plastic bags for additional protection. Once packed and closed, the container should be sealed with adhesive polythene tape.

The list overleaf is a guide in preparing a group medical pack (suitable for up to three people on trips lasting no more than five days). It can be scaled to suit the nature of the trip, taking into consideration the indicators listed at the start of the chapter. Note that with all medicines (prescription and non-prescription), their administration should be as directed by a qualified medical practitioner or follow any directions given on the packaging.

General Equipment

➤ 2+ pairs vinyl examination gloves

➤ Scissors

➤ Tweezers (fine point)

➤ Thermometer

➤ Splints

➤ Safety pins (various sizes)

➤ Disposable airway

➤ CPR mask

➤ Salt

➤ Electrolyte drink

➤ Notebook and Pencil

Wound Cleaning

➤ 36 surgical wipes

➤ Antibacterial soap

➤ 4 oz bottle of surgical scrub

➤ 2 surgical scrub brushes

➤ Povidone-iodine solution 10% (to provide antiseptic

➤ Irrigating syringe/bulb

➤ Tub of 100 cotton buds

Wound Dressings

➤ 2 large wound dressings

➤ 6 film dressings 6cm x 7cm

➤ 2 adhesive/cohesive bandages 5cm x 7m

➤ 15 packs of 5 sterile gauze swabs 5cm x 5cm

➤ 10 non-adherent dressing pad 10cm x 10cm

➤ 10 absorbent wound dressing pads 10cm x 10cm (sterile and non-sterile)

➤ 2 Fixomull dressing retention 5cm x 10m

➤ 2 Fixomull dressing retention 10cm x 10m

➤ 1 each of conform bandage 5cm, 7.5cm and 10cm

➤ 2 sachets of 4 Strips Steristrip 4 x 75mm

➤ 1 sachet of 6 Strips Steristrip 13 x 102mm

➤ Plasters (variety of sizes; larger sizes can be cut down)

➤ 1 roll of waterproof tape 25mm x 9.2m

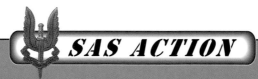

SAS ACTION

➤ Many SAS soldiers and military pilots carry a small tub of potassium permanganate crystals in their survival pack. When mixed with water they provide an all-round sterilising agent, antiseptic, mouth wash and anti-fungal agent.

Drugs List

It is difficult to provide a detailed list of drug treatments to include in your medical kit. On the one hand, the availability of certain medicines varies from country to country: obtaining prescription medicines in the UK, for example, requires a doctor's signature which can normally only be obtained when a person is ill or injured. In other EC countries such as Spain, however, many such drugs and antibiotic preparations can be freely obtained from pharmacies.

Also, the choice of drugs and medications carried should be tailored to fit in with the types of illness or injury you are most likely to encounter in your area of travel or for the type of activity you will be engaging in. For example, those travelling to the Far East will certainly require some form of protection against diarrhoea and mosquito-related infection. Therefore, the list below is offered only as a short guide to the many types of drugs and medications available.

WARNING

➤ Almost all drugs have some carry some side effect, although this is estimated to effect no more than 2 per cent of all users. These side effects can be mild to life-threatening and can include nausea, vomiting, dizziness, etc. Taking two or more different drugs at the same time can also cause a reaction, increasing or decreasing the effect of one or more drug. Drug toxicity, usually caused by incorrect dosage or accumulation, can be potentially dangerous when the body's mechanism is unable to eliminate the drug. As general rule pregnant women, children and those over 60 should not be given drugs unless a doctor proscribes them. In the wilderness, all efforts should be make to establish if a person is allergic to a specific drug; if no definite answer is forthcoming then it is up to the medic to evaluate the risk of possible side-effects against the prevailing illness or injury.

Antihistamine tablets
Used to control itching and various allergy symptoms. Some are also prescribed for controlling nausea, motion sickness and as a muscle relaxant.

Hydrocortisone cream (1%)
Used to treat allergic skin reactions and insect bite inflammations

Topical anaesthetic ointment
Gives localised numbing around skin surface areas needing treatment

Decongestant tablets
Provides relief from nasal and respiratory congestion and sinus inflammations

Antidiarrheal tablets

Ophthalmic ointment
Used for styes, mild eye infections, conjunctivitis and snow blindness

Antifungal cream
Used to treat athlete's foot, fungal infestions and sweat rash

Blister treatments

Pain control medication
Aspirin will relieve mild pain, headaches and reduce a fever. Ibuprofen 200 mg tablets are used to control inflammation, fever and pain.

Lip balm (with sunscreen)
Used to prevent chapping on lips. Moisturising cold sores

Sunscreen
Use high-factor cream or lotion tp prevent sun- and windburn

Insect repellant
Use those containing DEET

Antibiotic capsules or tablets
Used in the infection of wounds, the upper respiratory and chest infection. Always check with the casualty to see if they are allergic to penicillin.

Tetracycline antibiotic capsules or tablets
Used for bacterial infections of the chest and gut as well as for the treatment of tropical fevers. They can also be used for the prevention of wound infection.

In addition to the above, more specialised drugs (usually only available on prescription) can be obtained for the treatment and/or prevention of conditions such as malaria and other tropical diseases, and also of altitude sickness.